Reverse Arthritis and Pain Naturally:
A Proven Approach to an Anti-Inflammatory, Pain-Free Life

by Gary Null, Ph.D.

ESSENTIAL PUBLISHING

N. Palm Beach, FL
www.essentialpublishing.org

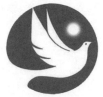

Essential Publishing, Inc.
378 Northlake Boulevard, Suite 109
North Palm Beach, FL 33408
www.essentialpublishing.org
(866) 770-1916

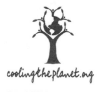

coolingtheplanet.org

PRINTED IN THE U.S.A.

This publication was printed by a Certified Green Printer in the United States of America, providing jobs for American workers. It was also printed, with the health of the environment in mind, on recycled paper and with vegetable-based inks, and Gary Null and Associates is planting more trees than were required to print this publication through *Cooling the Planet*.

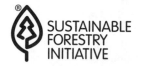

Acknowledgments

Creating a book of this magnitude required the untiring support of several individuals. I would like to express my gratitude to Nancy Ashley for her diligent research and editorial input. I thank Jeremy Stillman for his assistance verifying facts and editing text on several sections of the manuscript. I'd like to also thank Larry Hubbell for doing a meticulous job documenting our arthritis study. Finally, my special thanks goes to the top-notch staff at Essential Publishing, led by insightful publisher Morgéan Ó Conghalaigh, and his talented managing editor, Lynn Komlenic. Their steadfast dedication and brilliant creative input were crucial in bringing this project to fruition.

Table of Contents

Foreword

As a physician, I frequently read books and publications from both the conventional and alternative medical fields. I have found over the last few years that Dr. Gary Null's books carry an exceptional depth of research, knowledge and usable information, and *Reverse Arthritis and Pain Naturally – The Proven Approach to an Anti-inflammatory and Pain-free Life* is no exception. The importance of this new publication cannot be overstated given the frequency and severity of circumstances associated with arthritis, particularly in the U.S. The pain, disability, financial implications and loss of function associated with arthritis affect the human spirit and the quality of life for countless individuals, families and businesses in our country and around the world.

While conventional medicine, as we know it, focuses on symptom-based strategies for relief by patching the pain and inflammation with colorful pills and oftentimes ineffective surgeries that largely support the degenerative roots of arthritis, allowing it to slowly progress, this volume shines an extremely bright light on the highly effective alternative. *Reverse Arthritis and Pain Naturally* engages arthritis sufferers in the noteworthy mission of healing the cellular and molecular factors that *cause* this crippling disease. Most importantly, it employs us in a process of questioning and abandoning previously held assumptions about this disease as a *fait accompli* of aging.

As you consider the valuable information and testimonials within this book, you will discover that you can not only reverse your arthritis and enjoy a pain-free existence, but can be experiencing unprecedented health and vitality, substantially improving your odds of being free from chronic disease altogether throughout your life. Not only does Dr. Null postulate that the greater number of arthritis classifications are indeed related to "lifestyle" choices (diet, exercise, relaxation, stress-management, emotions, etc.), but he provides overwhelming evidence – both anecdotal and scientific – to the validity of this argument, shared by many physicians who work in the natural health world though, not surprisingly, an underwhelming few from conventional health care industries. Arthritis is an exceptionally lucrative business – more than $120 billion annually flows through a system of individuals as well as corporate and governmental entities who are more interested in protecting their status and wealth than in finding and supporting truly healing solutions, which requires a sincere investigation of the causes of the condition.

Dr. Null believes that unless we begin to understand and treat the very roots of the arthritic process, we will never be able to actually reverse it and attain functional improvement. And he is right. The ability of modern medicine to address symptoms is wonderfully effective for emergency and trauma situations, but is dangerously ineffective for lifestyle diseases. For these, you've got to look within for the causes before applying treatment from without, and this book is a major tool and guidepost for effective treatment.

What you will read irrevocably supports a new way of thinking about arthritis as eradicable *and* preventable in many cases. In support of already irrefutable evidence to the benefits of "clean living" in the avoidance of arthritis, Dr. Null tested his protocol in a four-week study – possibly the largest nutritional study related to arthritis yet – with overwhelming success. Nearly 80% of arthritis sufferers staying reasonably close to the recommendations realized improvements! This alone should tell us that something significant is missing in modern day arthritis treatment programs.

There is a reason why Dr. Gary Null has become one of the world's foremost authorities in the field of proper nutrition and how it positively affects health and healing. His findings and resultant publications are a beacon for the rest of us, and should be regarded with the highest esteem.

Before you discard your canes, walkers and pain relievers, however, it is wise to reflect on the *real* problem related to health – our persistence as humans to assign responsibility for our well-being to someone or something *outside* ourselves. In a matter of a very short time span in human existence, we have rendered ourselves useless in understanding and relating to the causes of health. If there is anything that could prevent you from being well, it is this. Consequently, the most important and provocative question in this eye-opening volume is related to our human nature rather than to arthritis itself. Why, queries Dr. Null, with all of the evidence in support of healthy eating and lifestyles, do we continue to make choices that cause us pain?

Reading and studying *Reverse Arthritis and Pain Naturally* is a required step for anyone wishing to understand and properly treat the human condition related to ill health, including arthritic conditions. If you contemplate what Dr. Null is saying here and adopt his recommendations, I am confident that you will find increased energy and vitality for life, and be well on your way to healing.

Dr. Null's explanation about the oxidative and biophysical core of the degenerative process, and the adversities brought about by improper social and cultural habits so widespread nowadays is particularly helpful. From the side effects of NSAIDs (non-steroidal anti-inflammatory drugs) to the adversities of unnecessary surgery, this book addresses and warns patients about common complications of irresponsible care, and advises them on how to regain one's own strength, power and influence in overcoming their ailment.

Throughout these pages, Dr. Null correctly provides crucial information on and directives for reducing inflammation – *the main cause of tissue degeneration in the human body*. He emphasizes the process of inflammation, oxidation and cellular decline, and accentuates the importance of omega-3, polyphenols and antioxidants in the prevention and repair process. *Reverse Arthritis and Pain Naturally* also draws attention to the fact that the adverse effects of free radicals and omega-6 can never be overstated, as these are major players in the process of cellular disruption and tissue destruction at the foundation of arthritis and bone deformity.

More critically, perhaps, is that arthritis is just *one* of the resultant illnesses linked to inflammation. Recent discussions in some of the most highly respected medical communities in the U.S. are now implicating inflammation in *all* disease, infectious and non-infectious alike, making this book a highly momentous, universal and widely relevant volume.

The *Nutrition Intervention Reverses Arthritis Symptoms* chapter is one of the highlights of the book and of tremendous importance, as is the chapter *Anti-Arthritis Supplements* – a terrific reference for patients, therapists, alternative medicine practitioners and physicians alike.

All in all, *Reverse Arthritis and Pain Naturally* clearly shows that treating arthritis with conventional medicine alone is both a flawed and hazardous approach. What we know in the medical field as alternative or complementary therapies must be accepted as viable, essential and even primary components for the eradication and prevention of any disease or illness. The evidence is obvious and indisputable. Without this crucial viewpoint and appropriate actions, expressed so thoroughly and distinctly by Dr. Null, we risk remaining victims to the limitations of an incomplete, imperfect medical system, and to our own ignorance.

I encourage you to take heed of the important calls within this text, and know that their foundation is real; I have seen it in my own practice time and again. With the proper combination of therapies, true healing and relief is available to just about any arthritis sufferer who wants it. Equally important to our success in eliminating this illness is our acknowledgment that arthritis is not predestined; it is preventable with a modicum of readily available education, proper guidance and committed action. This is something to celebrate!

To your health,
Daniel Nuchovich, MD
Medical Director, Jupiter Gardens Medical Center
Jupiter, Florida U.S.A.

Introduction

Thank you for taking this important first step in informing yourself about preventing and reversing arthritis naturally. By doing so, it tells me that you are ready to enhance your understanding and to inquire into the processes that will ensure you a happier, healthier life free from pain and arthritis. The guidelines and practices presented in this book will assist you and those with whom you share these valuable insights in dramatically improving arthritic conditions, and in many cases, in completely eliminating this debilitating disease. As you now begin to implement these proven natural solutions, you will not only prevent *dis*ease progression related to arthritis, *but be providing yourself with a powerful protection against many other illnesses as well.*

The first thing I want you to know is that I have seen firsthand just how serious and difficult it is to live with a painful and debilitating illness like arthritis. I wrote this book because I care about you and your well-being and want to see you and many others overcome the obstacles to healing. I also know how incredible life can be when we release our unhealthy habits and embrace health as a way of living. I can assure you, if you follow the guidelines I have provided, that you will begin to experience life in a new and possibly unimaginable way. Quality information is only part of what is needed in the creation of lasting health. In addition to the team of experts that I have called upon to fill this volume with important information related to your healing, I also need *one additional expert* to join your team – and that is YOU! As you read the valuable information herein from my colleagues and me about reversing and preventing arthritis, let yourself feel the truth of the words on a deep level, and then allow the intelligence within you to come forward and guide you. By taking the time to inform yourself, and then choosing to act on what resonates deeply with *you,* you will become your own health advocate, which is one of the greatest gifts you can give yourself.

You may find following through with these recommendations to be challenging at times. However, once you gain the clarity about what is really at stake – *the possibility of a long, healthy, vital and creative life* – you will, like so many thousands of others, find a way to pick up these healthy habits and continue to run with them. Ultimately, you will be the expert you've been waiting for, and an encouraging and supportive force in helping others address their health concerns powerfully. Caring for and sharing with others, after all, is what makes life truly rewarding and fulfilling.

The famous Greek scientist and physician *Hippocrates* (born in 460BC), considered by many as the founder of modern medicine, said – *"It is more important to know what sort of person has a disease than to know what sort of disease a person has."* He believed and demonstrated that the natural forces within us are the true healers of disease, and spent his life helping people understand all of the factors – physical and otherwise – in their lives that could be causing their *dis*-ease. Along with important information on fortifying the body with proper nutrition and exercise, he taught people how to care for themselves by providing compassionate, loving guidance, which is an essential aspect of healthy living.

Remember, as you take these important steps to correct the factors that caused your *dis*-ease, do so with an inspiring mix of gentleness and firmness. Be kind to yourself, yet be clear about what is needed for you to heal. Both are necessary for a happy and healthy life.

I have written *Reversing Arthritis and Pain Naturally* to give you the opportunity to consider and look more closely at the causes of arthritis and other diseases that you may be experiencing. I encourage you to reflect upon the important data contained herein regarding the efficacy of conventional medical practices in the treatment of arthritis versus those associated with natural arthritis treatment programs. When we don't have the complete story, we are vulnerable to participating in methods that may do far more harm than good. This is what I'm interested in changing with this book, and why I am introducing you to a new standard in the treatment of arthritis. After all, what is the use of getting a second opinion if it comes from the same paradigm as the first?

Having treated thousands of patients myself, and worked with hundreds of the nation's foremost physicians in the areas of arthritis and pain treatment, let me assure you that more harm is being done right now than good with today's modern practices. In spite of this, I can also confirm that if you are intentional and committed to living a healthy life, you *will* find your way, and this book *will* be a great asset to you on your journey back to Wellville.

Section I

The Pathology of Arthritis and Pain

- 1 -

Arthritis and Pain:
The Scope of the Problem

Surgeons in the United States are now replacing 500,000 knees annually along with 230,000 hips, and it is predicted that 67 million adults – a quarter of our adult population (an astonishing 1 out of every 4) will have some form of arthritis by the year 2030.

According to the Center for Disease Control (CDC) and the Arthritis Foundation, the disease known as arthritis is at the top of the list as the most common cause of disability in the United States, limiting the activities of a remarkable 50 million adults.[1,2] Surgeons in the United States are now replacing 500,000 knees annually along with 230,000 hips, and it is predicted that 67 million adults – a quarter of our adult population (an astonishing

1 out of every 4) will have some form of arthritis by the year 2030.[3] Globally, the picture isn't much brighter; an abstract published by the *National Center for Biotechnology Information*, reports that 200 million people suffer from rheumatoid arthritis alone.[4] Arthritis hasn't always been so prolific. So, what is fueling this crippling epidemic today? Most importantly, is it possible to prevent or reverse an illness that so many physicians and their patients believe to be irreversible? You may find the answers to these questions surprising, and not at all what you anticipated. You may also find it astonishing to learn that *currently accepted practices of treatment may actually be **worsening** your arthritis and **causing** other equally deleterious health challenges.*

To understand the complex matrix of the body and how it comes to the state of *dis*-ease called arthritis, we must also understand the intricate mix of factors of the world in which we are living today versus the times when arthritis wasn't so prevalent. Ultimately, our health is not separate from that of the environment in which we live, so comprehending physical disease – no matter the type – is as much a biological matter as it is a sociological, anthropological, psychological and ecological one.

Conventional wisdom holds that arthritis is oftentimes simply a part of aging and occurs in most humans over time due to wear and tear on our joints. But according to a 2005 National Health Interview Survey conducted by the CDC, two-thirds of people with arthritis were *under the age of 65,* including 300,000 children.[5] Such alarmingly high rates of arthritis among younger generations can be attributed to one underlying cause: our consumption of excessive amounts of highly concentrated calories and few viable healthy nutrients. In short, we are overfed and undernourished.

What are the inflammatory agents that are causing arthritis and other degenerative diseases in children and teenagers in particular? Simply put, the American diet of hot dogs, French fries, pizza, bacon, hamburgers, pastries, and soft drinks laden with high fructose corn syrup and caffeine. In effect, we have created – and continue to create – massive body pollution and a genuine five-alarm fire every time we eat or drink anything like this. As you will see, this type of diet is extremely low in antioxidants and phytonutrients, as well as chlorophyll, fiber and vegan sources of amino acids. So it is simply a matter of time until a child who eats this way manifests a disease, and merely a flip of a coin in terms of what disease it will be. We can be sure of this: children are manifesting lifestyle diseases, including arthritis, at younger and younger ages (the research proves it), and this won't change until we change.

> The fact is that we are not all destined to become arthritic with advancing age.

Exacerbating the problem is the fact that we as a population are becoming increasingly resigned to chronic disease as a "fact of life" – for ourselves and our offspring. While this couldn't be farther from the truth, this way of thinking is especially alive regarding arthritis. Millions of middle-aged Americans have resigned themselves to acquiring some form of arthritis in their lifetime; and, in fact, believe that there is nothing that they can do about it. So, at the first signs of pain, they typically respond by limiting their physical activities, taking non-steroidal anti-inflammatory drugs, and planning for an eventual joint replacement surgery.

But is this the only way to address arthritis? More importantly, is this the most intelligent way? By no means. The fact is that we are *not* all destined to become arthritic with advancing age; in truth most of us can avoid arthritis and in many cases even reverse it and its difficult and challenging symptoms. How, you ask? By simply following the guidelines provided within the pages of this book.

Arthritis can be said to be among the many lifestyle diseases plaguing today's Americans, along with cancer, diabetes, atherosclerosis, heart disease, hypercholesterolemia, dementia, and hypertension. The pathophysiology for all these diseases shares certain commonalities: we eat more, move less, and we don't consume foods that give us the necessary micro and macronutrients essential for optimal health. The toll from arthritis is significant: most arthritis sufferers refrain from physically challenging activities and one out of three arthritis sufferers experience work limitations. In fact, arthritis is a more frequent cause of activity limitation than heart disease, cancer or diabetes, contributing to the skyrocketing costs (both direct and indirect) associated with this disease – currently estimated at $128 billion in the U.S. each year.[6,7] Even more shocking, reports the CDC, is that among U.S. adults with arthritis, 47% also have *at least one other serious disease or condition*, including obesity, heart disease and diabetes.[8]

R esearch shows now that only one in four adults in America engages in any physical activity at all.

A Closer Look at the Problem...

As we have evolved rapidly into an ever increasingly immobile society – tethered to couches, electronics and motor vehicles – our bodies have followed. Except in the case of arthritis, the tether is some form of structural support for bodies that no longer move – a cane, a walker, a wheelchair, and in some cases even a new joint. Why are we progressing into a nation that cannot walk or move well? One of the reasons is that the structure of our living areas and buildings has changed markedly. Building designs of the early 1900s show that the majority of houses, churches, movie theatres and schools of the time had stairs. Apartment buildings in New York City from the early 1900s that were built with elevators nevertheless had steps outside leading to the front entrance.

Ranch-style living only became popular in the 1950s, and there were no elevators to access the New York City's subway system until the 1990s. The evidence is that we used to be able to move our bodies successfully under more challenging circumstances.

Furthermore, our society's transition from an agricultural and industrial society to a technology-based one over the last few decades has continued to change the way we move and live. Outside of the city, many of our ancestors used to farm; even if not farming for commerce, they very often had a family garden. Two-hundred years ago, 90% of the population farmed; today, it is less than 2%![9] Not only were they raising healthy, fresh foods for their families, they were getting regular daily exercise while doing it. Research shows now that only one in four adults in America engages in *any* physical activity at all. Instead, we drive our cars to the grocery store (or to the drive-thru window of a fast-food restaurant) to purchase food that has often been shipped by boat and by truck for several weeks before arriving on our tables. Typically, these foods are picked unripened, and are preserved with waxes and other potentially harmful chemicals in order to withstand damage from shipment and longer transport times, greatly diminishing their natural vitality and nutritional value. Is it any wonder that we are breaking down, growing weaker and more susceptible to the painful and debilitating side effects that accompany illnesses like arthritis?

Regrettably – and to make matters worse – the current medical paradigm avoids addressing the *root causes* of arthritis and other lifestyle diseases, which would necessarily require consideration of the aforementioned sociological influences, among others, on our health. Physicians rush in to apply the therapies they are most familiar with – drugs and surgeries – to the exclusion of more natural approaches for relieving pain and its causes. As my colleague Daniel Nuchovich, M.D., author of *The Palm Beach Pain Relief System* and Director of the Jupiter Gardens Medical Center, and the Jupiter Institute of Health, says "Most doctors rush into treating the symptoms of arthritis before even understanding the causes of it." This is simply not good medicine – a sentiment that is echoed by Norman J. Marcus, M.D., associate professor of anesthesiology and psychiatry at the NYU Langone School of Medicine, and author of *Freedom from Pain*, and *End Back Pain Forever*, who says: "Reducing pain is not enough with arthritis; we must also work to improve function, which requires a deeper understanding of all the mechanisms of pain."

As an example of the gross oversight of the effectiveness of traditional, common sense therapies, you will see evidence in a later section of this book that dietary therapy, including cleansing and fasting (used consistently since ancient times for decreasing the impact of accumulated toxins), is extremely effective in the reduction of arthritis symptoms, but also in the prevention and eradication of the disease itself. Yet, few American medical doctors are embracing this reality. It's truly astounding, when you think about it: how could such a simple and seemingly obvious aspect of good health not be universally accepted and included as a valid treatment? The same goes for sleep, for example. As a culture, we sorely underestimate the value of high-quality sleep in the prevention of and recovery from disease, including arthritis. According to the CDC, however, one-third of all American workers don't get enough sleep, and many who are sleeping enough hours are not getting quality sleep (tossing, turning, snoring, having disturbing dreams and waking up several times during the night to go to the bathroom etc.).[10] When basic physiological and emotional needs are lacking, the likelihood of developing diseases such as heart problems, depression, diabetes, and obesity (a direct cause of arthritis) increases. Still, these simple, common sense matters are often overlooked or discounted as immaterial by the medical community, when in fact they are directly related to *dis*-ease.

As always for us Americans, the emphasis is all too often focused on quick-fix strategies, including wonder drugs that create a false hope and expectation that we can miraculously continue living our lives exactly as we had been prior to the illness or disease. Instead of applying a thoughtful, intelligent, proven approach – like the one presented within the pages of this book – that includes paying attention to what we eat and maintaining a healthy weight through regular activity and exercise, we are offered medication for inflammation, diabetes, high cholesterol, and high blood pressure, along with surgical interventions, including joint replacement surgery. Do any of us want to keep our own body parts and live without carrying around bags full of pills? Sadly, only a very small percentage. The majority of us want the so called *magic bullet* – we are unaware of its dangers, including the false sense of security that it provides. Just take this pill or remove this part from your body and neutralize your pain, or so we are told. We continue to agree to expensive and largely ineffective medications and surgeries – in spite of feverishly escalating insurance costs – without thinking that we as individuals have any ability to affect what is occurring. As Dr. Nuchovich says, "Most people take a passive rather than active attitude with their disease, and expect the doctor to heal them. This almost certainly prevents them from actually getting what they want, which is relief from their pain." So the person that is still eating a terrible diet, drinking terrible beverages, or both, takes a handful of pills and does not feel the pain. But is the core problem addressed? No! But the number of people like you who are reaching out for quality information about your arthritis and pain, and willing to invest that invaluable and irreplaceable commodity – your time – to ensure that you join the ranks of the healthy and vital is rising.

While it is true that each of us has the ultimate responsibility for our health, and the ability to make changes with proper information and support, we also must recognize the powerful influence of the multiple billion dollar advertising and marketing industries, led by "masters of spin," on Madison Avenue. As a group, we are more significantly influenced by them than we realize. The good news is that we are also extremely influenced by pain, and will do most anything to be out of it. In order to break the spell that in one sense has been cast upon us, and – in another – that we have bought into, we need to ask ourselves a fundamental question, which is: *How do I want my life to be?*

Your answer to this question will guide you to take actions that support what you wish to see in your world. European countries, for example, do not permit advertising for pharmaceutical drugs on television. As a group, they recognize the ability of advertising to sway and manipulate their citizens. As such, they stay true to their convictions that these conversations must be guided by the medical community rather than by profiteering drug companies that will do anything within their power to sell their products. Lamentably, these organizations have a proven track record of misleading people to the point of causing very serious physical harm and even death. The fact that these predatory drug company executives invest repeatedly in promoting their extremely profitable products as beneficial while withholding empirical evidence to the contrary is perhaps one of the greatest ethical challenges of our time.

In order to resolve our country's enormous and continuously growing health challenges, including that of arthritis, we must begin to address our collective ignorance about the creation and maintenance of good health, including the psychology that keeps us trapped in belief systems void of common sense, consideration of natural order, and fraught with a perilous conviction to scientific authority. To the detriment of a truly enjoyable, fulfilling, pain-free existence, we pray for and allow "scientific advances" such as surgery and drugs to save us from the pain of poor judgment. Whether we over utilize technology because of its availability or because we feel entitled due to the exorbitant health insurance premiums we are paying, health conditions as serious as arthritis warrant an honest look at our inner processes, and the actions that they motivate.

If you have any doubt that we are on a path of self-destruction, it may surprise you to learn that a report by Milliman & Robertson, Inc.

in 1995 documented that up to 60% of surgeries performed in the USA were unnecessary![11] While this statistic is a somewhat dated, the issue continues to raise concern. An article that appeared in the *Washington Post* in August of 2012 (this year) reported that health policy researchers at the University of Michigan had recently looked at cardiology procedures done across the state and found that 43% (nearly half) should not have happened if surgeons had followed medical guidelines.[12] Pediatric Surgeon Catherine Musemeche wrote an article about unnecessary surgeries, appearing this past April in the *New York Times*, in which she related to children suffering from obesity: "We are taking out more gallbladders in younger and younger patients – by some estimates, more than four times the number of pediatric gallbladders are removed now than in 1990." She went on to say that "parents prefer to book the quick fix of the scalpel instead of the slow, but less invasive, route of lifestyle change."[13]

Indeed the number of surgeries is increasing, especially in outpatient, or ambulatory settings. The newsletter *Health Capitol Topics* reported that a statistical brief published by the *Agency for Healthcare Research and Quality* indicated that in 1980, 16 percent of surgical procedures were performed on an outpatient basis. This number grew to 57.7 percent in 2007.[14] There are a number of reasons for the growth in outpatient procedures, including lower costs as well as improved technologies and medical advances;

Physicians who obtained ownership of an ASC [Ambulatory Surgical Center] experienced a much higher increase in surgery use between pre- and post-ownership, in comparison to physicians who never became owners.

however, one of the primary reasons for the growth in the number of surgeries is the amount of money that can be made by the individuals – largely physicians – who own them. According to a report in *Risk and Insurance Magazine*, there were 2,200 Ambulatory Surgical Centers (ASCs) nationwide in 1996, and by 2009 there were 5,360, of which 83 to 88 percent were owned by physicians.[15] An article published by John M. Hollingsworth et al., in the April 2010 issue of *Health Affairs* indicated that there was a significant association between physician ownership of ASCs and higher surgery volume for selected procedures performed in those centers between 2003 and 2005; further, physicians who obtained ownership of an ASC experienced a much higher increase in surgery use between pre- and post-ownership, in comparison to physicians who never became owners.[16]

The trend is the same in elective surgeries related to arthritis. In 2005, at the 73rd annually meeting of the American Academy of Orthopedic Surgeons (AAOS), a research team from an engineering and scientific consulting firm Exponent Inc. presented a paper that projected the number of procedures for primary (first-time) total knee replacement would jump by 673 percent – from just over 500,000 currently to 3.48 million – in 2030, with the number of primary total hip replacements to increase by 174 percent – from 325,000 currently to 572,000 – in 2030. Furthermore, according to the authors, the number of revision surgeries was estimated to double in the next three years, by 2015, for total knee replacement and by 2026 for total hip replacement.[17]

More recently, *The Huffington Post* reported that knee replacement surgeries have doubled over the last decade and more than tripled in the 45 to 64 age group.[18] Hips are trending that way, as well. What's surprising, notes the article, is that it's not just related to obesity, but to our attempt to stay fit and avoid extra pounds. The surgeon quoted in the article attributes the increasing volume to what he calls "fix-me-itis," which is the mindset of "fix me at any cost, turn back the clock." While the article reports that knee replacements can last up to 20 years, it also says that because of the relative newness of this therapy the statistic does not take into account active younger baby boomers and seniors who plan on running marathons, skiing or playing tennis into old age.

Nonetheless, I want you to stop and think about this for just a moment...If many operations are unnecessary, then how is it that we (individuals and surgeons alike) are not entertaining a conversation of prevention versus the extremely painful and debilitating alternative of having our flesh cut open? Can you see just how insane things have gotten – where the majority of us will actually allow someone to perform surgery rather than embrace a lifestyle change? It's quite possible that this is the first time that you have heard such alarming statistics. Now that you are privy to the projections as well as the obvious conflict of interests, I ask you to reflect on this question: *What am I going to do about it?* An equally important question is, *What causes a nation to continue to engage so actively in obviously destructive and unwarranted activities, and why are we not considering that what we are doing may not be correct?* The answer is multi-factorial, but includes an understanding of human nature, as well as the programming that we are fed – and tend to believe – by interest groups (perhaps better named "conflict of interest" groups).

A Legacy of Bad Medicine

For more than 50 years, the American Medical Association (AMA) ruled over all medical health care in the United States. The American public was led by the AMA and the medical establishment to believe that all drugs, taken individually or jointly as in the case of multiple prescriptions, which generally apply to most seniors, could be consumed safely. Each year when the 20 leading causes of death were listed, heart attack, stroke, cancer, diabetes, etc. appeared at the top, with some variation. Nowhere

"**W**hat our research revealed was shocking: *the number one cause of death and injury every year for the past 15 years was American medicine.*"

– *Gary Null, Ph.D.*

was it reported that American medicine itself contributed to death or injury until a Harvard professor by the name of Dr. Lucian L. Leape took the time and energy to do an analysis. What he found was astounding: American medicine was the number one cause of illness. Commencing six years ago, I put together a research team of medical doctors and scientists, all of whom had extensive academic and research experience, and with myself, we set out to determine how severe a problem this was. To date, no one had analyzed and compiled all the published literature dealing with injuries and deaths caused by government-protected medicine. At the end of five years, we had a mammoth amount of research and what it revealed was shocking: *the number one cause of death and injury every year for the past 15 years was American medicine.* We surmised that from 550,000 to as high as 1 million people in the United States per year had died, and many millions more were injured, as a direct result of American medical practices. Causes of death ranged from adverse drug reactions (ADRs) and improper transfusions, to surgical injuries and wrong-site surgery; there were also suicides, restraint-related injuries or death, falls, burns, pressure ulcers, and mistaken patient identities.

I found this so incredible that I turned over the research we had completed to another friend who has a research background and was engaged in scholarship for further review. After three months of reviewing all the material, he said the conclusions we arrived at were all accurate. We then decided to take a further step and ascertain the areas of medicine that were not working effectively or safely but rather were increasing the likelihood of a negative outcome. We separated the data into categories such as cardiology, oncology, neurology, ophthalmology, urology, etc. What we found was that a high percentage of medical procedures for many conditions had *never* been established as safe and effective by a *gold standard test*, which consists of a long-term, double-blind, placebo-controlled initiative with crossover studies on human beings (clinical trials in which the study participants receive treatments in a random order). We are expected to accept on faith that these procedures are safe and effective simply because the doctors "believe" that there is proof.

Not surprisingly, we uncovered that behind all of this was an extraordinarily powerful pharmaceutical-industrial complex that exercises enormous influence over every aspect of the healthcare system. We learned that they work with the insurance companies and the for-profit hospitals utilizing massive lobbying campaigns to control virtually all federal regulatory agencies involved in healthcare policy, including the Food and Drug Administration (FDA) and the National Institute of Health (NIH). We also investigated the various tactics employed by them to dominate our entire U.S. public health service. The tactics included: placing their supporters, policymakers, physicians and scientists into key regulatory positions; controlling medical school curricula through lavish gifts and research grants; and making direct payments to physicians. Their power was further increased by extensive media campaigns; they are now – and were back then – one of the largest advertisers on television and radio, and in print media. As such, there is an enormous amount of self-censorship; no one from the media is going to expose them and risk losing their income flow. They also work to shape public opinion by funding front groups, think tanks and foundations. Well-known scientists and physicians go into the community and speak positively about them, but the public never knows they are really just hired guns pandering for Big Pharma.

Our report, *Death By Medicine*, is the most comprehensive review of the dark side of American medicine to date.[19] (See the *Death by Medicine* addendum in the back of this book for more a more in-depth explanation of this topic.) It is fully documented and referenced using only data gathered from mainstream sources. We sent our report to 7,000 individuals, including every member of Congress, every state legislator and governor, hundreds of journalists in the American media, more than one-hundred scientific journals, the National Cancer Institute, and the Library of Medicine. We waited and waited and waited; and not a single agency, lawmaker, or journalist touched the issue.

When you realize how many millions of Americans have died or been injured due to a lack of medical safety, or iatrogenesis (any adverse condition in a patient resulting from treatment by a physician or surgeon), surely you would think someone would discuss it, or hold a forum on it. But you'd be wrong. We offer several pages of this scientific article at the end of this book for your review, if you are inclined.

Substance Use and Abuse...

Tranquilizers and antidepressants keep you from feeling the pain of your life – as do marijuana, alcohol, and eating an entire box of chocolate in one sitting. It all works to *numb the pain in the moment* – be it physical, emotional, mental or spiritual. But as everyone learns eventually, compensatory behaviors (as they are called in psychology circles) provide only temporary relief. None of these momentary distractions sustain relief or resolve pain; and they all typically cause more damage. Aside from the fact that these substances are toxic, they don't directly deal with the underlying issues in our lives that many of us are avoiding.

This couldn't be truer than in the example of our prolific use of and reliance on drugs in this country – prescribed or otherwise – to manage pain. To start, the American Medical Association reported in 2011 that the annual costs associated with the more than 116 million Americans who suffer with pain were $635 billion – just shy of our $711 billion annual military expenditures.[20] This is a staggering statistic when you stop and think about it. According to Dr. Marcus, it may be surprising for you to discover that studies now indicate that in spite of the fact that we have more technology available to us, the number of people in pain has increased from 37.9 million people, or 15% of total US population, in 1990 to in 50 million people, or 22% of the total US population in 2009.

Regarding prescriptions, a report issued by the Centers for Disease Control in 2004 stated that half of all Americans took one pharmaceutical drug, with one in six people taking three or

> "...the Journal of the American Medical Association (JAMA) reported that prescription drugs taken as prescribed in hospitals are the fourth leading cause of death in the U.S. and Canada..."

more; furthermore, five out of six persons 65 and older are taking at least one medication and almost half the elderly take three or more[21]. This same report, issued again in 2009, concluded that the use of *three or more* prescription drugs increased for all age groups of males and females, and it is happening with increasingly deleterious effects.[22] A recent report issued in the *Journal of the American Medical Association* (JAMA) noted that prescription drugs taken as prescribed in hospitals are the fourth leading cause of death in the U.S. and Canada, after heart disease, cancer and strokes, causing about 106,000 deaths a year and over two million serious injuries in the U.S.[23] Even ordinary aspirin and ibuprofen are taking their toll with over 15,000 patients dying in North America annually.[24] A report by ABC News in April of 2011 about the use of prescription painkillers highlighted Vicodin, the most popular pain relief drug in the country at the time. IMS Health, the independent research and consulting firm who conducted the research for its annual survey of drug sales, reported that Vicodin prescriptions had grown dramatically from 112 million doses prescribed in 2006, to 131 million in 2011. The report went on to say: "Experts say most of those prescriptions are unnecessary." It also stated this astonishing fact: *The United States makes up only 4.6 percent of the world's population, but consumes 80 percent of its opioids – and 99 percent of the world's hydrocodone, the opiate that is in Vicodin.* In ABC News interviews, Dr. Thomas Frieden, director of the Centers for Disease Control and Prevention, pronounced "accidental overdoses from Vicodin and other narcotic pain relievers kill more people than car accidents in 17 states" and national drug czar Gil Kerlikowske declared, "the current culture of writing narcotic prescriptions for moderate pain, which began about a decade ago, needs to be changed and doctors need to be retrained. In the amount of education and training that doctors get, there was very little time, if any, in medical schools and other places to be devoted to understanding this [the highly addictive nature of opiods]."[25]

Our mounting dependence on pharmaceutical drugs in the alleviation of diseases and their symptoms, including arthritis and pain, is a relatively new phenomenon that has its roots in a 4,000+ year-old tradition of *herbology* – the study of herbs and plants that aid in curing illnesses and preventing disease. While manufacturers of pharmaceuticals say their products are "plant derived," what they don't tell you is that they are mostly comprised of synthetic chemicals (rather than actual plants), which affect our bodies in numerous harmful and still undetermined ways. Moreover, ingesting multiple pharmaceuticals creates an even more dangerous cocktail with truly unknown side effects. This is especially pertinent given that the majority of arthritis sufferers are plagued by other life-threatening diseases like diabetes and heart disease, and are taking additional medications.

While manufacturers are required by law to inform us of the potential risks and side-effects of their particular drug, they are not required (and hence do not seek) to test drug combinations. Those of our population who are taking multiple drugs are essentially walking Petri dishes. To complicate matters, in his treatment of people with pain and arthritis, James N. Dillard, M.D., D.C., L.Ac., Integrative Pain Management Specialist and former Director of the Rosenthal Center for Complementary & Alternative Medicine at Columbia University Medical Center, has found an association between high levels of pain and high levels of mercury toxicity. What this means is that pharmaceutical drugs are not likely the *only* toxic substances that your body is attempting to deal with if you have pain or arthritis. Heavy metal toxicity comes with our world's unprecedented levels of water and air pollution, contaminated seafood, as well as the widespread use of dental amalgams and vaccines containing mercury.

There is hardly a place on this planet that is not affected by the destructive ways of humans, and as individuals we are all affected in some way. Whether we are exposed to outgassing from new carpets or furniture, to pesticides and fungicides in our food and water, or to pollutants in our air, we are at constant risk. Unfortunately, there is plenty of research to attest to our challenge. When Bill Moyers filmed his special on chemicals called *Trade Secrets*, he volunteered to have his tissues biopsied. The test revealed nearly 84 distinct toxins.[26] On another note, recent testing of mother's milk found trace amounts of jet fuel, and testing of placentas exposed over 200 or so chemicals.[27] The truth is we are on toxic overload simply by virtue of the era in which we live.

Complicating the issue is that the government body (the U.S. Food and Drug Administration, commonly known as the FDA) formed to protect consumers and oversee the activities of Big Pharma has for decades been run by a board of directors comprised almost entirely of past and present CEOs and board members of the large multinational conglomerates it is meant to police. So the very board members that are regulating these organizations are deeply and incestuously tied to them – a classic example of inappropriate government/corporation collusion in direct conflict with consumer interest.

Today, with an estimated 13,000 pharmaceutical drugs on the market and a medical community beholden to the chemical giants that produce them – partly due to the astoundingly high costs of a medical education – we are unrestrained in both our use of and belief in these substances as "cure-alls."[28] Most of us have convinced ourselves that pharmaceuticals will help with just about everything, which couldn't be farther from the truth. In reality, only

Only one-half of the prescription drugs used actually work for the person who takes it.

one-half of the prescription drugs used actually work for the person who takes it.[29] Among cancer patients, the rate of ineffectiveness jumps to 75 percent, and antidepressants are effective in only 62 percent of those who take them.[30] If you're having trouble digesting the facts, just hear the words of Dr. James N. Dillard, M.D., D.C., L.Ac., "MOST of the patients I see with arthritis and pain are on the wrong medications." The number of drugs in production is even more astonishing when we consider the relative youth (less than 60 years) of the U.S. pharmaceutical industry and its governing body, the Food and Drug Administration (FDA). That it takes an average of 12 to 15 years to bring a new medicine from the laboratory to the pharmacy shelf at an average (and staggering) cost of $500 million per new medication leads us to a rapid understanding of our country's priorities in terms of "healthcare."[31]

By contrast, the ingested medicines of the "old days" consisted almost exclusively of plants and herbs – largely in whole form – and concoctions resulting from natural processes such as infusion, distillation, and fermentation that did not require the use of synthetic chemicals. "Medicines" included substances like alcohol and tobacco that are toxic to the human body when taken internally. However, with the exception of these, the larger percentage of our recent ancestors – even two generations ago – didn't have access to the chemically altering and addictive synthetic substances that are available today. They learned to deal with pain, disease and the stresses of life without them.

The Rise in Power of Drug Companies

How did these huge multinationals become so powerful, so quickly? Most of today's major pharmaceutical companies were founded in the late 19th and early 20th centuries; it wasn't until the 1920s and 1930s, however, with the discovery of insulin and penicillin, that pharmaceutical drugs became mass produced and more widely distributed. To its credit, penicillin – at the time called a "miracle drug" – forever altered the treatment of bacterial infections, and has saved countless millions of lives over the decades, the same can be said about insulin. Few doubted the benefits of drugs at this time; however, even fewer recognized their downsides and potentially destructive side effects. This is understandable in part because the earliest mass-produced drugs were so impressively death-defying that they earned pharmaceuticals their false reputation as "cure-alls" – *substances that are safe and keep us safe.* To our detriment, we have yet to release this belief.

Eventually, however, we learn that not all drugs are what they are cracked up to be. Opiates and amphetamines, as one example, were used primarily for the treatment of depression and pain in the early 1900s but were largely abandoned (because of their addictive qualities) for tranquilizers and antidepressants around the middle of the century. Ironically, the antipsychotic and antidepressant medications on the market today are equally devastating and addictive – if not more so – than the pharmaceuticals that preceded them. There are many more examples of the destructive nature of these substances (the ones related to arthritis are noted in this book); however, the critical point is that we as a populous assume that progression of time (often called "progress") is related to quality, which is not necessarily the case.

Nonetheless, the discovery of insulin and penicillin fueled a massive fire (that rages on to this day) within us to discover more life-saving substances. It also spawned our prevailing belief that health (and life itself) *depends* on drugs. So the industry and the people it serves march on intrepidly without considering two very important questions: Why do we find ourselves so ill in the first place? *And,* why have we all but abandoned natural, common sense practices used successfully for centuries in establishing and maintaining health? Supporters of the pharmaceutical model for the eradication and prevention of disease state that existing "miracle drugs" and the potential discovery of others are what motivate their steadfast alliance. However, there are many medical doctors, healthcare professionals and journalists today who believe that the industry was and still is propelled not by a benevolent and altruistic motivation to heal humanity, but by ignorance, greed and self-interest on the part of corporations and individuals. We will let you be the judge after considering all that is presented here.

As with most initiatives, there were problems early on; the pharmaceutical industry is no exception. It wasn't until the 1950s, in fact, that the industry demonstrated its recognition of the need for quality, consistency and accountability related to manufactured substances and adopted standardized scientific approaches in the creation and production of pharmaceuticals. While the Food and Drug Administration (FDA) was in existence at this time, it wasn't until the passage of the *Kefauver-Harris Amendment* in 1962 that the FDA gained any real strength over consumer products in the United States. This revolutionary amendment – enacted in response to the 1959 thalidomide tragedy, which resulted in birth deformities of thousands of European babies – required, among other things, that all new drug applications demonstrate "substantial evidence" of a drug's efficacy for a marketed indication, *in addition to* the existing requirement for pre-market demonstration of safety.[32] It was the beginning of our modern day FDA approval process, but one that also highlights the dangerous reality that human lives are at risk in these ventures, and even more so without proper regulation. See more about the risks associated with the current FDA approval process in the *Death by Medicine* addendum in the back of this book.

Why am I belaboring the history of pharmaceuticals, and what does this have to do with arthritis? The answer is quite simple: *If we don't understand the assumptions and prevailing beliefs underlying our modern medical system's largely failing approach to the prevention and eradication of lifestyle illnesses like arthritis, we will not question these assumptions and beliefs and address their shortcomings to the degree that is necessary to uncover truly effective solutions for what ails us. It is especially important that we confront the erroneous belief that pharmaceuticals and surgeries can "cure" disease and illness (which is false).*

It is helpful to consider the size of the problem, including the fact that the profits of the 10 pharmaceutical companies in Fortune's Top 500 are greater than the combined profits of the remaining 490 companies on the list.[33] Most naturopathic physicians today along with a select few conventional medical doctors are realizing this unpleasant truth: conventional medicine (surgeries and drugs) is the preferred treatment for arthritis sufferers, but alone cannot heal the degeneration associated with the disease. More importantly (because of its attention to symptoms rather than causes), conventional practices will most often lead to further deterioration. This is especially the case with osteoarthritis–

America's leading form of arthritis. As my colleague Dr. Nuchovich says: "I have seen time and again that the joint does not heal with conventional medicine; it gets worse. Integrative medicine, not allopathic medicine, offers a future – an improvement in function, a decline in the pain, and the possibility of healing." It is no secret that we as a nation are suffering tremendously by our diseases and by the treatments we are receiving in our attempt to address them. The pharmaceutical drugs prescribed now in grand excess, and purported to "prevent" and "treat" both the disease and their own side-effects, are especially egregious.

If we are to find and implement solutions that truly heal diseases like arthritis – rather than simply eradicating their symptoms – we must understand why they have come into existence in the first place, and learn how to distinguish between the causes and effects (i.e. symptoms). *Arthritis is a multi-factorial disease and unequivocally related to how we live*; a few intelligent cultures around the globe have known this over time, and chose more healthful options, including diet. As a result, their cultures experience less disease than others. The *Seven Countries Study*, pioneered by researcher Ancel Keys in the late 1940s, studied more than 13,000 men through 1981. It was the first study to explore associations among diet and diseases such as heart disease and stroke in contrasting populations, and it brought to light the advantages of the Mediterranean diet. The study, among other things, concluded that changing from a healthy, active lifestyle and diet to a less active one significantly increased the risk of heart disease – a leading lifestyle illness today. [34]

Recently, after a long career in research and policy-making related to the promotion of better health through greater consumption of meat, milk and eggs, T. Colin Campbell, Ph.D. published his similar findings in his avidly acclaimed book *The China Study*. The study, a 20-year partnership between Cornell University, Oxford University, and the Chinese Academy of Preventive Medicine, surveyed disease and lifestyle factors in rural China and Taiwan. The findings were

> "People who ate the most animal-based foods got the most chronic disease. People who ate the most plant-based foods were the healthiest and tended to avoid chronic disease."
>
> – *The China Study*

overwhelming: "People who ate the most animal-based foods got the most chronic disease. People who ate the most plant-based foods were the healthiest and tended to avoid chronic disease."[35] There are other examples of healthier cultures in our world: the Hunzas, the Bulgarians, and the Japanese of the Far East to name a few. Predictably, each of these cultures consumes a primarily vegetarian diet.

Perhaps even more relevant to the health of a culture is whether it is focused more on *function* and *health,* than *disease.* With an emphasis on health, a society's form and system of medicine would necessarily reflect activities proven to create health, including sensible measures of prevention. What we call "alternative" or "complementary" therapies in America, acupuncture and herbs for example, are traditional (or primary) therapies that have been in place and worked relatively well for a vast majority of people on this planet for thousands of years. Yet to our peril, our modern medical community mostly fails to acknowledge the importance of their role in our public health, and denies these and other contemporary "alternative" treatments as viable and critical elements of a treatment program. While our collective awareness is beginning to shift, the momentum is still very much more directed to disease management in our country than to creating vitality through natural, healthy living. The challenge associated with this line of thinking is that many suffering from arthritis come to these therapies too late in the game – after the damage has been done. When evaluating the data (the amount of money, resources and time, as well as the sacrifice in quality of life) associated with our modern treatments for arthritis, few would disagree that these treatments – on their own – have been an astounding failure. When we recognize this, and then juxtapose it with the obvious and time-tested benefits of natural and regenerative approaches for preventing and alleviating arthritis, anyone currently enrolled in a conventional treatment program would be hard-pressed not to immediately halt and make an abrupt 180-degree turn in their approach.

According to the CDC, today's newest generations are expected to die at a younger age than their parents.

An Earlier, Healthier Time

It was a much different time even 100 years ago. Life may have been considered by many to be more challenging overall, but it was likely healthier in many respects. Many of our parents and grandparents are or were first generation Americans. As such, it was not uncommon for them to be preoccupied in establishing a decent life for themselves. Many grew and prepared their own foods, sewed their own clothing, walked to work or church, chopped their own wood, and relied on their community. While poverty and hardship was commonplace, and culturally there was far more emphasis on and threat to survival, people were more active and typically spent much more time out of doors and with one another.

Lifestyles have changed radically because of so-called *modern conveniences* and we are paying the price. As members of one of the most affluent and developed societies in recent history, we are, ironically, developing lifestyle diseases at alarming rates. Have you ever stopped to think about all the riches and benefits we have in this country compared to our recent ancestors and people in other countries, and then wondered how it is possible that we could be so shockingly unhealthy?

Lifestyle diseases like arthritis are slowly eroding our personal health, as well as the health of our families and our nation. They are making us more sedentary, more somnolent, more prone to infection, more likely to miss work, less likely to participate in our communities and to volunteer, and much less likely to *enjoy our lives*, which for the first time in recent history are becoming briefer. According to the CDC, today's newest generations are expected to die at a younger age than their parents. Instead of achieving a longer lifespan than our parents, we are now extremely unlikely to live as long as they did.[36] Others of us, sadly, will literally die *before* our parents due to our poor states of health, affected in large part by the declining health of our food, air and water quality. This, indeed, should tell us that something is very wrong with the way we are thinking about health, and how we are going about establishing and maintaining it.

While we have so much more technology and information available to us than our parents' generation did during their lives, we also have ever-increasing levels of environmental toxins, including heavy metals, PCBs from plastics, and PAHs from petroleum products that have infiltrated every one of us, affecting our chances and those of our offspring for healthy longevity. Do we really believe that we can survive the damages of our highly industrialized, commercial, chemical-laden world without appropriate and vigorous interventions?

As a nation, we are not, on the whole, paying attention to tell-tale signs of declining health, nor have we become a group that is willing to look more deeply for the causes of this decline, and take responsibility for changing it on a wholesale level. Conservatively speaking (because the numbers are growing daily), two-thirds of all Americans are overweight. Globally, we have the highest rates of obesity (a common cause and effect of arthritis) with more than one-third of U.S. adults (35.7%) and approximately 17% (or 12.5 million) of children and adolescents aged 2 to 19 affected.[37] The CDC reports that the frequency of obesity is a whopping 54% higher among people with arthritis compared to those without.[38] We are in fact digging our own graves with our forks, our largely sedentary lifestyles, and the stress of our continuous attempts to maintain unsustainable structures and systems; and we still do not understand the degree of impact on our health of so called *technological progress*. Whether it is the known and unknown effects of electromagnetic pollution from our everyday use of appliances like microwaves, mobile phones, smart meters, I-pads and computers, or the deaths caused by radiation or texting while driving, it is clear that our technologies are not only harming us, they are killing us too. Technological advances, almost universally heralded as the hallmark of our generation, remain to be seen if they are, indeed, forwarding us as a society and species, or simply moving us backwards. It is an imperative inquiry as we become more and more isolated from one another and the natural world. With declining health, longevity and now happiness – based on recent studies – there is no clear evidence yet that we are indeed progressing.[39]

> "My team conducted a four-week study with people currently suffering with and being treated for arthritis. *Eighty percent (80%) of participants realized improvement in arthritic conditions.*"
>
> – *Gary Null, Ph.D.*

The Bright Spot in All of This...

There is good news, however, and it is this: you *can* make a shift, you *can* change your life for the better, and you *can* prevent and reverse arthritis and live a potentially pain-free life without drugs and surgeries. For many decades now, I have worked to influence millions of people to adopt the practices outlined in this book. I have seen remarkable transformations in people, and can attest to the benefits that occur when people are not only *willing* to take action, but when they *actually do* take action. In preparation for writing this book, my team conducted a four-week study with people currently suffering with and being treated for arthritis. *Eighty percent (80%) of participants realized improvement* in arthritic conditions – a reduction in pain and swelling, and increased mobility – as well as key health-related markers like better sleep and improved mental clarity with my protocol. These are astounding results, and I am hopeful that they are all you need to hear to proceed with incorporating the healthy protocols provided in this book.

This book not only provides you with a much clearer understanding of the causes of arthritis, including its chief instigator – *inflammation* – but it describes the deleterious effects of relying solely on a system of medicine founded and entrenched in pharmaceutical and surgical interventions to manage this largely lifestyle disorder. We describe the differences, after you have been diagnosed with arthritis, between entering treatment from the allopathic versus the naturopathic side and the probable outcomes with both. You also gain valuable insights on the prevention and reversal of arthritis using ancient as well as ultra-modern "alternative" therapies proven to alleviate arthritic conditions.

Equally important is my discussion about returning to a more natural way of living, which includes food and supplement guidelines and recipes, suggestions for proper exercise and movement, the importance of pure water and hydration, recommendations for reducing your exposure to environmental toxins, tools for stress reduction, and the examination of the mental, emotional and spiritual aspects of disease. Whether you suffer from arthritis currently or are determined to avoid it, by the time you have incorporated the valuable guidelines in this book, you will be well on your way towards reversing your arthritis and regaining your health.

Perhaps of greatest importance, you will know that you are not alone in your struggle. Thousands of others like you are challenged daily by arthritis but are making these valuable, lasting changes that are improving their bodies, their health and their lives in unprecedented ways. Because we understand the challenges associated with change, we offer suggestions on how to implement and sustain your new habits. As you will see, our mental and emotional process surrounding disease is a key determinant in whether we overcome disease to lead a healthy life.

It is a radical and subversive notion to take responsibility for your health and your life. It is also, undoubtedly, an immensely powerful, liberating and intelligent one because when you know how to heal yourself, you are *truly* free. Then, you can live happily and healthfully for whatever time you have on this extraordinary planet. Furthermore, when you undertake the process of becoming healthier and happier in life, you become a beacon of inspiration for others along the way, and quickly discover something that I have known for quite a while now: helping our fellow human beings is one of the most satisfying endeavors in life. Yes, there will be naysayers and challenges on your road to recovery, but the extraordinary feelings and results you will experience after only a few weeks on this program will serve as both your testimony and your motivation for adopting the practices outlined here as a way of living.

I am grateful that you have taken this decisive step, and welcome you as a part of our global group dedicated to eradicating arthritis and pain, but also to embracing the crucial rediscovery of healthy living.

- 2 -

What is Arthritis?

We are told that arthritis is the result of the overuse of joints; this is actually not correct.

Arthritis is a group of conditions which affect the joints, causing stiffness, pain, and restriction of movement. Literally translated as *joint inflammation*, from the Greek word "arthron" (joint) and the Latin word "itis" (inflammation), arthritis consists of essentially100 different types of conditions, the most common of which are osteoarthritis, rheumatoid arthritis, and gout.[40] Joints are possibly the most critical part of human anatomy related to physical movement; it would be impossible for us to perform even the simplest of movements without them.

Brilliantly constructed of a complex, synergistic mix of tissue, bone and fluids, joints connect and allow the movement of two bones in tandem while preventing them from rubbing against one another and causing damage. The tasks literally weighing on our joints from day to day are tremendous. Not only are joints essential for body movement, they must also withstand the immense compressive forces – including body weight – that occur during movement.

Our joints get a little help from our bones. A fibrous capsule surrounding the ends of our bones creates a space which allows the juncture of the bones to withstand these potentially large forces. However, the joints must have protection of their own. Tissue lining the joint capsule, known as the synovial membrane, secretes synovial fluid to nourish the cartilage in and around the joint, and cushion it from adjoining bones. Whenever there is damage to one or any part of the joint resulting in stiffness, pain, and a loss of movement, we call it arthritis.

Osteoarthritis

Osteoarthritis (OA) is the most common type of arthritis in the United States and, in addition to gout, is directly caused by poor body mechanics and lifestyle choices. A chronic degenerative joint disease, osteoarthritis currently affects some 27 million Americans – a number that is increasing independent of our aging population.[41] Before age 55, a greater percentage of men are troubled by osteoarthritis, but after age 55, most osteoarthritis sufferers – 60 percent – are women.[42] There are two types of OA – *primary* and *secondary*. Primary osteoarthritis is generally associated with overall weakening and degeneration of weight-bearing joints. Secondary osteoarthritis is a result of an injury, trauma, or surgery, or the long term effects of obesity. The joints most commonly affected are knees, hips, fingers and shoulders, although any joint can develop arthritis in the case of injury or physical stress.[43]

Osteoarthritis involves the loss of articular cartilage, the formation of bony spurs at the joint margin (osteophytes), inflammation of the synovial membrane, and changes to the subchondral bone. As cartilage in the joint breaks down, bones start rubbing against one another, initializing an irreparable cascade of structural breakdown. The friction of bone on bone causes fragments of bone and cartilage to break off and rub against the bones, creating further irritation and pain during movement. Mobility becomes increasingly restricted and pain increasingly intense; this usually leads to less activity, which worsens the situation, as a lack of physical activity causes our muscles to weaken and decline. Over time, osteoarthritis can also damage ligaments and meniscus membranes, making it difficult to do daily activities including work, play sports or even just walk from place to place without struggle and pain.[44,45]

Onset and progress of arthritis is usually slow. Symptoms of pain, stiffness, and restricted function don't usually present themselves until after age 40, and become more prevalent with advancing age. We are told that arthritis is the result of the overuse of joints; this is actually not correct. In reality, the wear and tear associated with arthritic conditions comes from using only a *fraction* of the joint's actual range of motion; so it is literally the underuse of joints that causes arthritis. Let me explain. Active joints are generally healthier than inactive joints; but utilizing a joint improperly causes numerous problems. Movement that is tense and uses the body in an unbalanced way, places needless stress on certain areas of the body, including joints. Likewise, stronger muscles can compensate for weak or underdeveloped muscles, straining some unnecessarily while permitting others to atrophy. This creates a torque effect on joints, damaging the joint as well as the surrounding muscles while causing a reduction in the circulation of joint fluid. As the muscles continue to tighten, the capacity of joints to use their full range of motion is compromised.

Improper movement can also distort posture, which contributes to an unequal distribution of weight and pressure on all parts of a joint. If only a small part of a joint is forced to absorb all of the pressure of impact, the result is damage to the cartilage.[46] If we habitually stand on one leg, carry a heavy bag exclusively on one shoulder, sit with our legs crossed, perform the same exercise routine over and over, and spend much of the day sitting in a slouched position, we are contributing to the limited mobility of our joints and therefore predisposing ourselves to arthritic conditions. In fact, as you will see, it is our own abuse of our bodies that leads to the breakdown of our joints, and the onset of arthritis. On the positive side, there are numerous forms of exercise and therapies to assist us with proper and beneficial movement.

Signs and Symptoms

Joints affected by osteoarthritis usually ache or become painful or stiff first thing in the morning, or during physical activity or shortly thereafter. They may also be stiff after periods of inactivity. There can be a loss of range of motion that makes certain movements difficult or impossible. For example, someone with arthritis can lose the ability to kneel or get up off the floor. As movement becomes restricted, balance tends to diminish from lack of use. The stiffness can often lead to joint swelling, which includes pain. Without intervention, the situation worsens and joints become increasingly more dysfunctional and incapable of allowing the body to move as it was intended.

While most laboratory tests will not show changes that result from osteoarthritis, researchers have found that there will be an elevation in an enzyme called C-reactive protein (CRP), which is a marker for inflammation. CRP levels in the blood have been shown to correlate well with CRP taken from the synovial fluid in the joint from patients with osteoarthritis, and there is growing evidence that elevated CRP levels are associated with severity of the clinical course (medical treatment) of osteoarthritis.[47]

Cartilage

Cartilage is a flexible connective tissue consisting of three types, hyaline, elastic, and fibrocartilage, which are found throughout the body. In joints, hyaline cartilage lines the bones, providing a cushioning effect to the joints, helping to distribute forces during repetitive pounding movements like running or jumping, and acting like a shock absorber. If any aspect of the complex cartilage system breaks down, it can result in the degeneration of the entire joint. Because cartilage lacks a blood supply, it is a relatively vulnerable tissue. In arthritis, pressure on cartilage from movement and excessive weight bearing, along with chronic inflammation, can lead to thinning and damage.

R esearch shows that some NSAIDs [such as aspirin] actually damage cartilage and worsen joint function, even while relieving pain.

Standard Osteoarthritis Treatment

The mainstay of osteoarthritis treatment has been a reliance on non-steroidal anti-inflammatory drugs or NSAIDs. Each year over 70 million prescriptions are given to arthritis sufferers in the United States for these drugs, not counting the 30 billion over-the-counter NSAIDs sold annually. The most common NSAIDs are: aspirin, celecoxib, diclofenac, etodolac, fenoprofen, ibuprofen, indomethacin, ketoprofen, ketorolac, nabumetone, and naproxen.[48] These drugs interrupt the normal function of an enzyme known as cyclooxygenase, and lead to a reduction in pain and swelling that can greatly improve movement. However, the problem lies in the fact that not only are these drugs *not* benign, but research shows that some NSAIDs actually damage cartilage and worsen joint function, even while relieving pain. The use of NSAIDs halts one part of the inflammatory process that results in the breakdown of cartilage, but it also halts the companion part of the process which allows for the reformation of new cartilage.[49] So if we follow our doctor's advice and take NSAIDs regularly, we could end up damaging our joints in the process.

NSAIDs are so ubiquitous in our culture that we reach for a bottle at the least sign of discomfort without even thinking that they might do us harm. But NSAIDs first and foremost are extremely harsh on the gastrointestinal tract and can cause GI bleeding, impaired cardiac function, asthma and ulceration. It has been estimated that 15-20% of patients taking NSAIDs regularly for chronic disorders such as rheumatoid or osteoarthritis experience adverse GI events, and 100,000 Americans are hospitalized each year for resultant gastrointestinal bleeding. In elderly patients, this risk increases to five times that of control groups not taking these drugs. While few studies have examined NSAID-related mortality, evidence suggests that there are at least 16,500 deaths per year due to complications from NSAID use in the U.S.[50]

More deadly than gastrointestinal ulceration and perforation, however, are the cardiovascular effects of the newer COX-2 inhibitor class of NSAIDs such as Celebrex and Vioxx. These drugs selectively target the activity of COX-2, a cyclooxygenase enzyme that plays a central role in the inflammatory process. While they were designed to cause less harm to the GI tract than the older generation of NSAIDS, COX-2 medications are significantly more likely to cause heart attack, stroke, and sudden death – a rather poor tradeoff. Most egregious in this class of drugs is the story of Merck's Vioxx, the blockbuster NSAID that sold billions of dollars' worth of medication while increasing the risk of heart attack by 500%. It is estimated that in its five years on the market, Vioxx killed 60,000 people and caused heart attacks in at least 100,000 more. In fact, the damage was probably much more severe than that. After Vioxx was removed from the market in 2004, there was a sudden and marked drop in cardiovascular mortality of 50,000 people within six months.[51,52]

While Merck clearly knew, even prior to the FDA approval of Vioxx, that it presented a dangerous cardiovascular risk, this potential was minimized during the approval process. Eventually, however, the sudden and substantial increase in mortality in arthritis sufferers who took Vioxx forced Merck to withdraw the product. Despite all the evidence demonstrating the damage to individuals caused by Vioxx, Merck's deep pockets have allowed it to fight every lawsuit brought by victims and their families, and thus far they have not been forced to pay retributions for much of the multi-billion dollar profit they made from the blockbuster anti-inflammatory.[53]

So what about the other COX-2 inhibitors, like the number two seller, Celebrex? In 2004, a study of the drug found that 400 mg a day more than doubled the risk of heart attack and stroke, and 800 mg a day increased the risk of heart attack and stroke by greater than 300%.[54] In April 2005, after an extensive review of data, the FDA concluded that it was likely that there is a "class effect" (meaning all drugs in a category exhibiting similar behavior) for increased cardiovascular risk for all COX-2 NSAIDs, and recommended that Pfizer withdraw Bextra, another popular COX-2 inhibitor. Furthermore, they recommended that all COX-2 prescription NSAIDs be revised to carry a box warning highlighting the potential increased risk of serious adverse cardiovascular events, in addition to the warning about life-threatening GI bleeding which was already in bold on the box.[55] Nevertheless, despite safety concerns, these drugs remain on the market and are still used by hundreds of thousands of people each day.

While there is no drug that can restore cartilage, nutraceutical strategies have shown success in preserving cartilage in cases of osteoarthritis. Most notably, glucosamine has provided symptomatic relief and has slowed loss of knee cartilage in numerous studies.[56] Although still in their infancy, regenerative therapies are a potential rising star in the quest for non-invasive therapies. One of the current techniques showing promise for the future allows cartilage cells to be harvested from the knee, grown in a culture, and then re-implanted, causing cartilage to regenerate. Autologous Chondrocyte Implantation (ACI), as it is known, is performed at some of the major medical centers throughout the country, and can result in a return to functionality without knee replacement surgery.[57] A recent prospective study on patients who underwent ACI after having no success with conventional cartilage treatments found that 76% of all those surveyed experienced clinically significant improvements after a 2-year follow up.[58]

Joint Replacement

Knee and hip replacement surgery has become an extremely popular treatment alternative for arthritis sufferers, especially in the case of rheumatoid arthritis. An astonishing 25% of all rheumatoid arthritis sufferers undergo total joint replacement, with 25 percent of those requiring an additional arthroplasty (surgical repair of joint) within one year and a whopping 50 percent within seven years. As I mentioned earlier, each year the numbers of these types of surgeries increase, and they are offered as a miracle cure for degenerating joints. The reality falls a bit short of a miracle, however. Joint replacements currently last 12 to 25 years before they stop functioning well and need to be replaced themselves – not nearly the lifetime of one's own knee or hip.[59] Additionally, there is no data, yet, on the success of joint replacement strategies for individuals who remain assertively active (tennis and running for example) into their later years; the data drawn so far simply relates to older individuals with below average to average activity levels.

Despite the fact that new technologies are making life easier for patients with artificial joints, mechanical implants often limit their ability to run, jump, or engage in other high-impact activities and competitive sports. Titanium knees are significantly heavier

An astonishing 25% of all rheumatoid arthritis sufferers undergo total joint replacement, with 25 percent of those requiring an additional arthroplasty (surgical repair of joint) within one year and a whopping 50 percent within seven years.

than one's own knee, and range of motion can be significantly curtailed. A healthy functioning knee has a range of motion of 120 degrees to 150 degrees while a mechanical knee tops out at 110 degrees, with only slightly more than half of patients reporting improvement in stair climbing.[60]

The failure rate in hip replacement is significantly higher than that in knee replacement, most recently since the advent of metal-on-metal artificial hips. Metal-on-metal hip joints are a recent innovation developed to address the needs of younger arthritis sufferers who want more strength and durability from hip replacement. Thought to be more suitable for an active lifestyle, these implants have turned out to have significant adverse events previously unseen with the original metal-plastic hip implants. Concerns about the safety of metal-on-metal devices were raised in April 2010, when a British health agency published a report about problems with these devices. The journal warned that patients with a metal-on-metal hip replacement could experience damage to the soft tissue at the site of the implant caused by loose metal fragments, which could cause pain or other symptoms and require additional surgery.[61] The FDA found further, in May 2011, that because of the loose metal fragments, patients could experience problems such as blindness, deafness, thyroid problems, anemia and kidney failure due to elevated levels of cobalt or chromium in the bloodstream. The Food and Drug Administration asked 21 manufacturers of metal-on-metal hip implants – including DePuy Orthopaedics, Stryker, Zimmer, Biomet and Wright Medical Technology – to conduct a safety review of these products, and some of them have already been removed from the market.[62, 63]

There are other concerns, in general, regarding hip replacements. The National Institute of Medicine reported that the most common problem to occur soon after surgery is hip dislocation.[64] Since the artificial ball and socket are smaller than the body's normal ball and socket, the ball may become dislodged if the hip is placed in compromising positions. Artificial hips are not meant to bend beyond 90 degrees, so activities that we take for granted like tying shoe laces must be modified post-surgery.[65] There is also the risk, albeit low, of infection and blood clotting just after surgery, which can lead to death. After initial recovery, the typical complication is an inflammatory reaction in the area that causes cells to eat away some of the bone, causing the implant to loosen. In this case, revision becomes necessary.[66]

Additionally, there are several medical conditions such as severe neurologic, emotional, or mental disorders, severe osteoporosis, and obesity that could limit the possibility and success of replacement surgery.[67] Rehabilitation after surgery is critical for all patients, and the ability for and success of rehabilitation is closely related to other health factors such as muscle strength and adequate circulation, which involves vascular and heart health. Without significant therapy, many patients are worse off after the surgery than they are prior to the procedure.

Rheumatoid Arthritis

Rheumatoid arthritis (RA) is an autoimmune disorder whereby the immune system, which is designed to protect our health by attacking foreign cells such as viruses and bacteria, instead attacks the body's own healthy tissues, specifically the synovium, the thin membrane that lines the joints. This immune process causes membranes around the joints to become inflamed, and release enzymes that cause the surrounding cartilage and bone to wear away. Scientists estimate that about 1.3 million people in the United States have rheumatoid arthritis, and this number is on the rise.[68] Furthermore, according to the World Health Organization (WHO), RA affects 0.3–1.0% of the general population globally, and is more prevalent in developed countries.[69] The disease occurs in all racial and ethnic groups, but affects two to three times as many women as men.[70] This is largely due to the fact that women go through perimenopause, menopause and post menopause, all of which cause substantial alterations in hormone levels that tax the immune system, leaving women more vulnerable to this form of disease.

Up to 50% of all rheumatoid arthritis sufferers become unable to work, and have a higher mortality rate than the general population. Unlike with osteoarthritis, rheumatoid arthritis typically begins in middle age, often in the early 40's. Children and young adults, however, can also be affected.[71] Rheumatoid arthritis is typically not just diagnosed on physical symptoms alone, but also through blood testing, which usually reveals an elevated rheumatoid factor as well as antinuclear antibodies, which are special types of antibodies whose presence suggests a predisposition to autoimmune illness.

Individuals with rheumatoid arthritis often experience pain, swelling and stiffness in their joints, especially in the hands and feet. As a secondary symptom to inflammation, fluid builds up in the joints, causing painful swelling that can eventually result in bone erosion and joint deformity. Early rheumatoid arthritis tends to affect the smaller joints first – particularly the joints that attach fingers to hands and toes to feet. Periods of increased disease activity, called flares, alternate with periods of relative remission, when the swelling and pain fade or disappear. As the disease progresses, symptoms often spread to the knees, ankles, elbows, and hips.[72] In most cases, symptoms occur bilaterally, in the same joints on both sides of the body.

Rheumatoid arthritis can make activities of daily living extremely difficult as the hands and fingers become increasingly compromised, and any type of movement – lifting, grabbing, opening and closing lids, and carrying items – becomes difficult and painful. Persistent inflammation, joint swelling, and limited mobility result in stretching of tendons, ligaments and joint capsules with subsequent development of joint instability, decrease in muscle mass, and decrease in strength and mobility. Rheumatoid arthritis patients, especially those that suffer from severe cases, run a higher risk of infection, lung disease, heart attack and heart failure.[73,74] Progressive loss of function starts to develop early in rheumatoid arthritis. About one-quarter of those with rheumatoid arthritis develop nodules – called Heberden's nodes – that grow under the skin, usually close to the joints. Additionally, fatigue, anemia, neck pain, as well as dry eyes and dry mouth can also occur in individuals with the disease. Increased catabolism (metabolic breakdown) caused by rheumatoid arthritis raises energy expenditures, which leads to weight loss (referred to as rheumatoid cachexia). Eventually, rheumatoid arthritis results in severe disability and death for its sufferers.[75]

Up to 50% of all rheumatoid arthritis sufferers become unable to work, and have a higher mortality rate than the general population.

Why is it that some of the symptoms of rheumatoid arthritis appear unrelated to joint health? The answer is that inflammation in the body from any source extends throughout the entire body, negatively impacting all cells. It is a complete myth that an inflammatory attack is tissue-specific when, in fact, the contents of your blood are reaching every cell in your body. For example, the pro-inflammatory cytokines produced in the body after eating a well-done hamburger may cause a person's knees to swell. Even though it appears that the knees are the only affected part, the cytokines are also, for instance, contributing to the buildup of toxic amyloid plaque in the brain, and impairing normal liver function. By the same token, a lack of knee swelling after eating the hamburger doesn't mean that someone isn't being affected by inflammation on the fundamental level. This is the dangerous thing about inflammation. Let's say every time you eat a hamburger your knees don't swell. Does this mean that your joints are *not* being affected, or that your brain or liver are fine? The answer is, "no." Chronic inflammation is problematic for everyone, and it affects *every* body; it just may take years or even decades until the damage is so severe that you've reached your tipping point. Unfortunately, by this time you have a verifiable, diagnosable condition, and you are long past the moderate response stage – you are, in reality, at the end stage, which is different, but your doctor cannot tell you so. What we do know is that one person may end up with arthritis or fibromyalgia, and someone else with diabetes or cancer, all of which are diseases of inflammation.

The Rheumatoid Arthritis-Osteoporosis Link

Osteoporosis translates directly from Greek as "porous bones," and is a disease of the bones that leads to an increased risk of fracture. In osteoporosis, bone mineral density (BMD) is reduced, bone microarchitecture deteriorates, and the amount and variety of proteins in bone are altered.[76] Studies have found an increased risk of bone loss and fracture in individuals with rheumatoid arthritis, and hence a direct link to osteoporosis. The inflammatory process associated with rheumatoid arthritis causes bone destruction, particularly in areas immediately surrounding the affected joints. The pain and loss of joint function caused by the disease often results in inactivity, further increasing the likelihood of osteoporosis from lack of weight-bearing activity. Likewise, the glucocorticoid medications commonly prescribed for treatment of rheumatoid arthritis trigger significant bone loss.[77] Of special concern, as previously mentioned, is the fact that women, a group that is two to three times more likely than men to have rheumatoid arthritis, are also statistically at increased risk for osteoporosis.

Standard Rheumatoid Arthritis Treatment

There are many standard treatments for rheumatoid arthritis, which are meant to halt the immune response and relieve pain and swelling, but unfortunately none actually cure the disease, and all of them can inflict significant harm. These include NSAIDs, corticosteroids, and disease modifying antirheumatic drugs (DMARDs).[78] Treatment regimens vary, and can include a combination of numerous different drugs designed to interrupt the inflammatory process. NSAIDs, as previously discussed, carry the risk of gastrointestinal ulceration and perforation, along with heart attack and stroke. Corticosteroids have been linked to diabetes, fatty liver disease, Cushing's syndrome, osteoporosis, truncal obesity, and muscle wasting, the partial or complete wasting away of muscle tissue. DMARDs include a variety of chemotherapy drugs (methotrexate, azathioprine, cyclophosphamide, cyclosporine), sulfasalazine, gold, antimalarials, antibiotics, and the new biological drugs (Humira, Enbrel, Remicade), which can cost more than $2,800 a week. These drugs have a wide range of side effects that can result in a variety of serious ailments, such as malnutrition, osteoporosis, liver damage, diabetes, increased incidence of infection, and further degenerative diseases.[79]

Furthermore, in order to stave off the osteoporosis that so often accompanies rheumatoid arthritis, many doctors are prescribing bisphosphonates, drugs such as Fosamax and Boniva, which interfere with the naturally-occurring elimination of bone tissue through a process known as bone remodeling (breakdown and regeneration).[80] The theory behind these medications is that if bones are *prevented* from breaking down as a normal course of their function, then they can't lose bone mass. This is the fallacy – but it's also the danger related to humankind's ignorance and arrogance that we can somehow outsmart nature. In fact, if bones cannot function as they were designed, which includes bone remodeling, then they, in fact, become more brittle and are more likely to break. Bisphosphonate use has been specifically linked to the death of bone tissue through a process known as avascular necrosis, and to neck fractures, esophageal cancer and atrial fibrillation. Women are now cautioned not to stay on these drugs for greater than five years.[81]

One has to ask why neither the FDA nor prescribing physicians ever questioned what could possibly be the value of a drug that could be taken only for a maximum of five years because of safety reasons. In the meantime, a patient's life could undoubtedly be worsened through increased fracture and infection rates. The only ones who benefit in this deal are the pharmaceutical companies who have already made billions of dollars from this shady venture. The reason I am advancing these difficult questions and reflections is that it is necessary for you to know about the danger that you face in choosing pharmaceutical intervention for inflammatory conditions like arthritis. If you know the dangers, you have the opportunity to choose safer methodologies in the treatment of these challenging illnesses.

As of 2011, more than eight million American adults are now affected by gout; and the number is on the rise.

Gout

Gout, also called gouty arthritis, used to be known as the disease of kings because it was most commonly found in those who could afford to eat an opulent diet rich in meat, fat and alcohol. The affliction is widely portrayed in 18th century caricatures of enormously fat, well-to-do people with swollen feet and ankles. Gout seemed to have almost faded into history during the early part of the 20th century, but as Americans are becoming more overweight, and as cheap food has made large quantities of meat and fat available to the masses, gout is making a strong comeback. People like to think of gout as an inherited condition; if it is in our genes, there really is no reason to consider changing our lifestyles, they think. But the incidences of gout have more than doubled over the past twenty years! This stunning increase points more directly to the fact of the increasing girth of our nation's population than to our genetic predisposition to weakness.

As of 2011, more than eight million American adults are now affected by gout; and the number is on the rise. Gout is the most common form of inflammatory arthritis in men, affecting approximately 3.4 million men as of 2004. Interestingly, gout is no longer a condition that strikes men alone. Recent studies have shown that the incidence of gout in women has also doubled over the last 20 years, especially in the post-menopausal age group. Below age 65, the ratio of male to female gout sufferers is 4:1, but after age 65 the ratio drops to 3:1. There is some suggestion that estrogen helps reduce levels of uric acid, which appears to protect younger women.[82]

Gout is a type of inflammatory arthritis that is caused by the buildup of uric acid crystals from metabolism of excessive amounts of purines. While purines are produced naturally by the body and have many crucial functions, including the conversion of food to energy, they are damaging in excess.[83] When purines break down they form uric acid, which is normally eliminated from the body through the kidneys. For gout sufferers, however, uric acid cannot be eliminated properly and builds up in the bloodstream. When uric acid reaches high levels in the blood, it spills out into the tissues, forming uric acid crystals, which cause irritation and inflammation, and can result in loss of function. An accumulation of crystals in the joints and soft tissues can be excruciatingly painful and incapacitating. Because this most commonly affects the big toe, foot, or ankle, gout can significantly interfere with walking and mobility in general. Chronic inflammation of gouty arthritis can also cause fluid accumulation, further hampering movement and causing even more widespread pain.

. The evidence suggests that gout is strongly associated with metabolic syndrome – a group of health conditions characterized by central obesity, insulin resistance, high blood pressure, and blood lipid issues that also have been correlated with development of diabetes, heart disease, and premature death. While researchers have speculated that gout contributes to obesity and hypertension, and that an excess of uric acid may contribute to other conditions such as heart attack, stroke, or diabetes, it appears more likely that gout is not the cause, but rather another consequence of significant weight gain and increased waist circumference.[04]

Standard Gout Treatment

Treatment for gout includes the use of NSAIDs and colchicine to reduce the inflammation and help with the pain of acute attacks, along with drugs to block the production of uric acid such as allopurinol. Since 2009, newer drugs such as Uloric, which block uric acid production, have entered the market. More drugs are now in the pipeline since it has been recognized that the pool of gout sufferers is on the rise.

The good news is that gout is actually one of the most preventable and treatable forms of arthritis because the causative factors are predominantly tied to lifestyle. Although one cannot control naturally-occurring purines in the body, gout can be reversed (and prevented) first and foremost by simple dietary modifications – avoiding the foods most linked to the development of uric acid. High levels of meat and seafood consumption, in addition to alcohol consumption, are associated with an increased risk of uric acid and, therefore, gout. Dietary changes including the elimination of alcohol, and foods with high concentrations of purines such as meat products, especially internal organs such as liver and kidney, as well as beef, poultry, pork, lamb, fish, seafood, and meat extracts such as bouillon and gravy, are essential. Unfortunately, this basic, common-sense recommendation is frequently omitted by health care professionals in favor of advocating pharmaceutical intervention. This is due, in part, because of the supposed difficulty of restricting alcohol and certain foods, but also because many health care professionals erroneously believe that eliminating vegetables that are high in purines will help. While plant foods contain purines and some online resources and outdated dietary sources advise against eating lima beans, asparagus, beans, lentils, peas, and spinach, current scientific evidence not only shows that the consumption of these plant foods does *not* lead to an increased retention of uric acid but that these foods are the best defense against developing gout and maintaining a normal weight.

All in all, the single-best way to avoid or reverse gout is to adopt a program of dietary excellence. This would mean adopting a plant-based vegan diet that eliminates all animal foods, processed foods, and foods high in fat, and includes foods rich in antioxidants, phytochemicals, and natural anti-inflammatories such as omega-3 fatty acids, ginger, and turmeric. Physical activity is also an important part of avoiding or reversing gout as is losing excess pounds, especially around the waistline.

- 3 -

The Causes of Arthritis

Our immune systems...were not meant to be chronically under siege like they are today – by diets that are no longer rich in anti-inflammatories, a flood of environmental pollution, extreme stress, lack of regular and sufficient exercise and sleep, and punishing overweight and obese conditions.

What causes arthritis? Arthritis is a multi-factorial disease, meaning that there are many causes. Few would argue that the chief culprit is inflammation; however, even fewer of us understand the causes of inflammation, which will be discussed thoroughly in this chapter. One thing is certain: in order to prevent or alleviate arthritis, we must be actively involved in creating and living an anti-inflammatory lifestyle.

Inflammation

Inflammation is a normal defense process of our immune system that protects us against infection, wounds and other trauma. It causes invading pathogens to be killed and initiates tissue healing. For most of human history the inflammatory response has been tightly regulated by our own immune system, so that it can efficiently destroy an invader while not harming the body. This self-regulatory process functions via negative feedback mechanisms whereby anti-inflammatory mediators are secreted to quell the natural inflammatory process. Our immune systems, however, were not meant to be chronically under siege like they are today – by diets that are no longer rich in anti-inflammatories, a flood of environmental pollution, extreme stress, lack of regular and sufficient exercise and sleep, and punishing overweight and obese conditions. Today, inflammation is the common link in the vast majority of lifestyle diseases. If something happens to cause the inflammatory process to become excessive or chronic, regulatory feedback cannot work successfully and severe damage can occur.[85] Studies have shown that chronic inflammation leads to osteoarthritis, rheumatoid arthritis and gout, along with a host of other diseases including metabolic syndrome, atherosclerosis, lupus, diabetes, asthma, multiple sclerosis, non-alcoholic fatty liver syndrome, and Crohn's disease, to name a few. And while osteoarthritis is often categorized as a degenerative joint disease, there is ample evidence that its roots also are in inflammation.[86]

So what is fueling this increase in inflammation? First and foremost is our greatly increased consumption of fats – of all types – over the past 40 years: saturated, trans, polyunsaturated and monounsaturated fat consumption is up 63% since 1970.[87] Fats aren't all bad, of course, and the body requires some to work properly. Unfortunately, healthy fats such as those from avocado, nuts and seeds to name a few are the least likely to be consumed in the Standard American Diet (SAD), which we will be discussing in more detail later in the book. In reality, we must consume these healthy fats to form our cell membranes and hormones, without which we couldn't live. But most of the fats we require to live can be made by the body except for two polyunsaturated fatty acids: the essential fatty acids linoleic acid (an omega-6 fatty acid) and alpha-linolenic acid (an omega-3 fatty acid). In Section III, we will discuss healthy sources for these nutrients. Aside from these two fats, we don't require additional fats in our diets, and certainly not at our current levels of consumption.[88]

Polyunsaturated fatty acids, such as omega-6 and omega-3, play a vital role in the composition of all cell membranes. They maintain homeostasis for correct membrane protein function and influence membrane fluidity, cell signaling, and gene expression. There are many other omega-6 and omega-3 fatty acids that occur in fats aside from the two that we need, and these fats need to be in proper proportion to each other for optimal health. The ratio of omega-6 fatty acid to omega-3 fatty acid should be in a range of 1:1 or at most 4:1. Due to our dietary changes over the past four decades, however, our current ratio is 10-20:1. Why is this a problem? Researchers have discovered that the cascade of inflammatory mediators begins with something called arachidonic acid, which is in the omega-6 family. Arachidonic acid is found in all animal-based fats; and, as it is metabolized, it is broken down into factors which cause inflammation, constriction of the blood vessels, and a tendency for blood to clot. Omega-3 fatty acids do the opposite and actually help calm or halt inflammation. Because both omega-6 and omega-3 fatty acids are broken down by the same enzymes; there is a competition between the two. As long as the ratio of omega-6 to omega-3 is 4:1 or less, the enzymes preferentially metabolize omega-3 over omega-6, which keeps inflammation at bay. If a diet is high in meat, dairy, and other animal-based foods, however, then production of omega-6 takes over, and the overwhelming response will be the production of factors which cause inflammation, which is the case with the Standard American

Diet. In order to stave off inflammation, it is necessary to consume a diet high in omega-3 fatty acids, which are found in abundance in green leafy vegetables, chia seeds, flax seeds, and walnuts. Our Western diet, with its heavy emphasis on processed foods, is high in vegetable oils, animal products, and saturated fats, and low on green leafy vegetables, nuts and seeds. This leads to progressively higher levels of omega-6 fatty acids, which cause the diseases of inflammation: arthritis, cardiovascular disease, obesity, diabetes, inflammatory bowel disease, rheumatoid arthritis and cancer.[89]

> M ost commonly used mono- and polyunsaturated vegetable oils are just like animal fats, and they are rich in harmful omega-6 fatty acids.

Over the years, our fat intake has changed from primarily saturated animal fat sources to vegetable oils – the consumption of which has increased 225% from 1970 to 2004![90] Although we think of these oils as harmless, most commonly used mono- and polyunsaturated vegetable oils are just like animal fats, and they are rich in harmful omega-6 fatty acids. Peanut oil, safflower oil, sunflower oil, corn oil and olive oil all have omega-6:3 ratios of over 13:1.[91] A better choice of plant-based oil, with more abundant omega-3 fatty acids, can be found in walnut oil and flax seed oil. Even with the better oils, however, in order to maintain good health, we have to stop using them as if they were water. All oils, no matter what the type, do have one thing in common: 120 calories per tablespoon. So drowning your food in walnut oil will not lower inflammation and reduce arthritis if you become obese in the process. Consider other omega-3 sources: omega-3 fatty acids can also be found in most green leafy vegetables, grains, legumes, non-green leafy vegetables, fruit, wild-caught salmon and oily, cold-water fish, walnuts, flax seeds, and chia seeds.[92] Although fish are touted as an excellent source of omega-3 fatty acids (because their oil contains the long chain omega-3s EPA and DHA), fish don't synthesize omega-3 fatty acid themselves, obtaining it instead from eating green vegetation. We are fully capable of converting short chain omega-3s to long chain omega-3s ourselves if we just consume enough of them, and EPA and DHA can also be obtained directly from blue green algae. Farmed fish are not a good alternative because they do not have access to a natural diet and, therefore, tend to have oils high in omega-6 fatty acids, not to mention all the other toxic realities of farm fishing. When fish are maintained in small confined spaces, unable to eat a natural diet or get away from their own waste products, disease results. They become heavily burdened by infestations of sea lice and injuries from other fish, and develop illnesses from living in excessive bacteria. As a result, they are treated with large amounts of toxic chemicals to combat lice and other pathogens, as well as antibiotics to fight bacterial infections and hormones to foster growth. In stark contrast to the promotion of fish as a healthy inflammation-fighting food, farmed fish are so ill and contaminated that they can only cause inflammation and should not be consumed under any circumstances.

Oxidative Stress

Oxidative stress is a complicated concept. The body produces defensive factors from oxygen molecules that have the capacity to kill invaders such as bacteria, viruses, and cancers. These defensive factors are called *reactive oxygen species*, and include peroxides, oxygen ions, and free radicals. Problems can develop in the elimination of these reactive oxygen species, especially if they remain active past the time needed to kill the invader. In this case, they will start to damage the body itself, which is referred to as *oxidative stress*. Like inflammation, oxidative stress is the result of a normal biological defense process designed to protect the body from harm. The reactive oxygen species are produced to attack and kill pathogens, but can cause severe damage to proteins, lipids, DNA, and all components of the cell. Damage to the cells can also disrupt normal communication between the cells, resulting in disease. Oxidative stress can initiate an inflammatory response, which in turn sets the stage for chronic inflammation and the development of arthritis.[93]

The main antioxidant that our body uses to eliminate free radicals and other reactive oxygen species once they are no longer needed is *glutathione*. Glutathione is a protein molecule that is synthesized in the body from three amino acids: glycine, cysteine, and glutamate. Even though we can make glutathione ourselves, we don't necessarily make it in sufficient quantity to eliminate all the reactive oxygen species that occur. When glutathione is deficient, illness and chronic disease can result. Studies have shown that consuming synthetic glutathione is *not* effective in correcting a deficiency. What does work, however, is supplementation with foods that contain the building blocks to assist the body in making glutathione. Foods such as broccoli, Brussels sprouts, cabbage, cauliflower, garlic, onions, avocado, asparagus, and walnuts have proven to be effective. There are also useful supplements, such as N-acetylcysteine and SAMe (S-adenosylmethionine).[94]

The Link between Environmental Toxins & Oxidative Stress

A key contributor to oxidative stress and disease is environmental toxicity. We live in a different world today than even 50 years ago, so it is imperative that we understand this and change our thinking about how to remain healthy. In order to overcome arthritis, we must carefully consider other aspects of our environment and make appropriate changes. From ergonomics, to body mechanics, to the toxins that we are exposed to and ingest on a regular basis, we face an uphill battle in clearing the obstacles that lead to degradation to restore and maintain health.

There are toxins not only in our air and water, but in our foods as well. The importance of consuming organic food is especially clear for those facing arthritis and other chronic diseases. The simple facts that organic foods are not genetically modified, and do not have the level of pesticides, fungicides, herbicides and other deleterious chemicals that conventional produce contains, mean from the get-go that you are creating less inflammation in your body by consuming them. Additionally, heavy metal exposure from sources such as dental amalgams can cause many problems in the body including liver toxicity, loss of brain function and joint pain.

It is also essential not to underestimate the challenges associated with food allergies. Allergic responses trigger an inflammatory response; so regular consumption of foods considered to be highly allergic to the human body (corn, wheat, dairy, peanuts, etc.) can be especially damaging. If you know you suffer from allergies of any kind, it may be helpful to secure an allergy test to determine the full array of allergens that may be sensitive to, and eliminate those allergens as best as possible to reduce inflammation.

Cleansing and detoxification, a practice employed by numerous cultures over time, is extremely effective for ridding the body of excess toxins, and for preventing and eradicating illness. While the practice is gaining in popularity here in the U.S., it is a relatively foreign concept to many Americans. It is, however, an essential consideration for anyone facing a chronic disease. The body is miraculous; it has built-in intelligence to create homeostasis (balance), and therefore health; but with so many assaults, from so many sources, its abilities become compromised. It is up to us to help our bodies as much as we can so that it can do the job it is meant to do. If you desire to undergo a cleansing and detoxification program, it is recommended that you seek guidance from an experienced, reputable professional.

Acidity and the Standard American Diet

Not enough can be said about the importance of a balanced pH. The body is such a phenomenal thing, operating mostly on its own without our knowing. Most people don't know that one of the body's primary functions is to maintain a balanced pH; our life – in fact – depends on it. Unfortunately, because the Standard American Diet is so acidifying, it creates a tremendous load on our bodies, which predisposes us to disease and illness. While this topic is vast, suffice it to say that it is critical to obtain the majority of our nutrients from alkalinizing food sources such as fresh raw vegetables and fruits. You will find additional information about alkalinizing foods, as well as lists of the most alkaline-forming foods in Sections II and III.

Of all the animal proteins, meat merits special attention in the pathogenesis of arthritis because research has shown that greater meat consumption is associated with a higher prevalence of degenerative arthritis in both men and women.

Meat

Of all the animal proteins, meat merits special attention in the pathogenesis of arthritis because research has shown that greater meat consumption is associated with a higher prevalence of degenerative arthritis in both men and women. The reason for this appears to be twofold. All meat is a rich source of arachidonic acid, which has a key role in starting the inflammation cascade, which leads to pain, swelling, dysfunction, and eventual joint destruction. An interesting study of the Seventh Day Adventists in California sheds some light on this finding. Seventh Day Adventists are the group with the longest life expectancy in the United States, and they experience significantly less morbidity and mortality from chronic diseases compared to the rest of the population. The religion emphasizes a healthy lifestyle, including healthy eating. As such, they encourage a plant-based vegetarian diet and discourage the eating of meat, and the use of alcohol, drugs and caffeine. A long-range study was done on the incidence of osteoarthritis in the Adventist communities among vegetarians vs. those who consumed meat, poultry and fish, where smoking and other factors were controlled for. The results showed significantly less arthritis among those Adventists who maintained a meatless vegetarian diet. More arthritis was seen in those who ate meat only once a week or less than in those who abstained completely, and the most was seen in regular meat eaters.[95]

The second major reason for meat's role in the development of osteoarthritis is that meat eaters tend to be heavier than non-meat eaters. A meta-analysis in 2001 of 36 studies of women and 24 studies of men showed that vegetarians had significantly lower weight (−7.7 kg for men and −3.3 kg for women; $P < 0.0001$ and $P = 0.007$, respectively), and a 2-point lower BMI than their meat-eating counterparts.[96] After adjusting for lifestyle and dietary factors, the differences in BMI remained significant, suggesting a direct correlation between low BMI and low meat consumption. These findings were supported by those from the European Prospective Investigation into Cancer and Nutrition (EPIC) study, which showed the highest BMI in the "meat-eaters" group and the lowest BMI among vegans. Meat consumption, therefore, appears to lead to weight gain, which can result in arthritis due to increased pressure on joints.[97]

Countries having the highest dairy product intakes also have the highest fracture rates.

Bone Loss

Osteoporosis, which we discussed earlier, is a potentially disabling disease in which the bones deteriorate and easily fracture; and it can exacerbate the debilitating effects of arthritis. The disease affects 25 million Americans, 80 percent of whom are women.[98] Much is made in the news and advertising about the risks of osteoporosis and the need for women to increase dietary calcium through the consumption of dairy products, but this advice runs counter to the evidence. In fact, countries having the highest dairy product intakes also have the highest fracture rates. Studies show that per capita consumption of animal protein is associated with a higher risk of hip fracture in women over 50 years of age, and consumption of vegetable protein is associated with a low fracture risk.[99] Eliminating animal protein altogether and maintaining a diet high in vegetables brings the risk down to an almost imperceptible level. Osteoporosis is significantly more prevalent in Western industrialized countries, where the ingestion of dairy products is at its highest compared to parts of the world where there is little or no access to dairy, or other animal, products. The reason for this appears to be the highly acidic nature of animal protein. In fact, in addition to providing a framework for our bodies, bone also functions as a reservoir for calcium when it is needed as a buffer. Animal protein such as meat or dairy is highly acidic, and ingesting it causes the body to respond quickly to reestablish a normal pH that is slightly alkaline. The primary alkaline buffer in the body is calcium, and it can be quickly obtained from the bones. The body's ability to buffer the acid caused by starvation or a high meat diet provided a survival advantage during hunter-gatherer times, because the consequence of acidosis was rapid death.[100] But now, we are eating so much animal protein that our bones are literally dissolving. Experiments have demonstrated that when the body is challenged with a dietary acid load from meat or dairy, the kidneys excrete calcium in the urine, and there is a drop in total bone density. Even a small drop in pH (increase in acidity) causes a tremendous increase in bone *resorption*, which is the process by which bone is broken down and minerals are released, resulting in a transfer of calcium from bone fluid to the blood. While it is critical to keep the acidity level of the body within an acceptable range, the downside is that when calcium is removed from the bones for this purpose the bones become less stable. Without some method to rebuild the bones, this calcium loss is a problem that becomes progressively worse, leading to osteopenia and osteoporosis. This excessive stimulation of bone turnover also causes an unnatural increase in bone *remodeling*, which is the replacement of old bone cells with new. While remodeling is a natural process, and occurs in adults at a rate of about 10% a year, excessive remodeling can itself weaken the bones and lead to the development of osteoporosis.[101]

Another major contributor to osteoporosis is the ingestion of carbonated cola drinks. These drinks contain a high level of phosphoric acid, resulting in a pH of only 3.0 for cola. The pH of the body is maintained at 7.35 to 7.45, and the human kidneys can only excrete urine with a pH of 5 or higher, so it then becomes necessary to pull calcium from the bones in order to neutralize a single cola drink.[102]

Why Else Are We Developing Arthritis at Such an Alarming Rate?

The number one factor contributing to the development of arthritis today is obesity – 54% of arthritis sufferers are obese, and recent studies show that both arthritis and obesity are increasing in prevalence in the U.S. In 2003, 38 states reported 30% of their population as obese, but in the ensuing six years, by 2009, the number of states reporting obese populations of 30% or more had risen to 48! Almost every state in the nation![103] According to the CDC, 35.7% of American adults were obese as of 2010, compared to 23% in 2005 and only 12% in 1990.[104] The rise in obesity has led to increased stress on all joints, but the knees are especially affected because these are the joints that carry most of the body's weight. It is estimated that each extra pound of weight actually adds four additional pounds of pressure to the knee joint.[105] A 2008 study on lifetime risk of knee osteoarthritis showed that obese participants had a lifetime risk of 60% compared to 30.2% in normal weight participants.[106]

I n 2003, 38 states reported 30% of their population as obese, but in the ensuing six years, by 2009, the number of states reporting obese populations of 30% or more had risen to 48!

America's Obesity Epidemic

There have been alarming headline news stories recently about the obesity crisis in America. We are the fattest nation on earth and getting fatter. Statistics show that two thirds of Americans are overweight and, conservatively speaking, at the very least one-third of the American population is now obese – defined as a Body Mass Index (BMI) of over 30. An advocacy group that relies on government figures for its projections announced this September that it expects an alarming 50% or more of the population in the vast majority of states to be obese by 2030![107]

The group also anticipates associated medical costs to increase $48-$68 billion over the U.S.'s current costs of $147-$210 billion annually, and that costs from loss of productivity could rise from $390 billion to $580 billion yearly.

According to a study published on Medscape Reference, approximately 21-24% of American children and adolescents are overweight with another 16-18% obese. The prevalence of obesity is highest among specific ethnic groups, said the report, and The National Health and Nutrition Examination Survey (NHANES) indicated that obesity is increasing in all pediatric age groups, in both sexes, and in various ethnic and racial groups, including whites. While there are many factors, including genetics, environment, metabolism, lifestyle, and eating habits that are believed to play a role in the development of obesity, NHANES researchers believe that less than 10% are associated with hormonal or genetic causes.[108] Moreover, a provocative new study just published in the *Journal of the American Medical Association (JAMA)* reports a connection between the Bisphenol-A (BPA) chemical used in plastic food packaging and childhood obesity.[109] Bisphenol-A (BPA) is an organic compound that is widely found in a variety of plastics, including plastic containers labeled with the number 7, plastic food wrap, cash register receipts, and the resins that coat the majority of metal cans. It is so prevalent in today's products that it is even in refrigerator shelving, water pipes and flooring. Since 1991, scientists have known that BPA is an endocrine disrupter that mimics the hormone estrogen; they also know that exposure to environmental estrogens during critical periods of development actually encode the body for obesity in the future. The damaging effects of the chemical include weight gain, changes to sex organs and their functions, increased tumor formation, hyperactivity, neurotoxin effects, and early onset of puberty. Because of the health risks to babies and young children, BPA has been banned in the production of baby bottles. The JAMA study found that children with the highest levels of BPA chemicals in their urine were twice as likely to be obese as those with the lowest.

Unsurprisingly, we even have a new category of obesity, which is now large enough to merit its own name: *morbidly obese*. This group, with BMIs of over 40, has shown the most striking increase from 1988-2008, and as of 2011 an estimated 6.6% of American adults can be classified as morbidly obese.[110] Many of the pundits are blaming the high levels of carbohydrate consumption linked to fast foods while the opposite camp is blaming high levels of fat. The debate is prolonged, endless and viewed by many health professionals as pointless. Americans have allowed themselves to become mindless victims of the food industry, aided and abetted by the surgical, pharmaceutical and advertising industries as it

A provocative new study just published in the *Journal of the American Medical Association (JAMA)* reports a connection between the Bisphenol-A (BPA) chemical used in plastic food packaging and childhood obesity.

relates to health in particular. As the food products we eat continue to weaken our health and make us sick, we run more and more for pharmaceutical and surgical interventions, keeping the entire system in place. If we ever realized that the key to maintaining health is within us, these industries would crumble from lack of business. But, we find ourselves in a complex, immense maze of unfounded beliefs, unsubstantiated actions and psychological deception (including misperceptions of our own inherent inadequacy and powerlessness) that are preventing us from asking truly intelligent questions and formulating appropriate plans. The situation is literally killing us. Unfortunately, speaking the truth invites lawsuits, so few in the know are willing to state the obvious. Why is it that only one-third of us are capable of maintaining a normal weight? We are obese because we consume high quantities of calorie-dense food products all day long and burn few if any calories in regular physical activity. It is all answered by simple arithmetic: calories in are dwarfing calories out.

Things are so out of control that state and city governments are getting involved; most – at a minimum – are considering a tax increase on sugary sodas, candy and fast foods; others are showing their concern about growing obesity rates by taking more aggressive actions. In addition to an already adopted ban on trans-fats earlier this year, New York City Mayor Michael Bloomberg plans now to ban sugary drinks and fatty foods from NYC hospitals, and to limit sodas and other sugary drinks, sold at restaurants, delis, sports arenas, food carts and movie theaters regulated by the city health department, to 16 ounces. This unprecedented but highly celebrated move to curb obesity is being lauded by other health-seeking lawmakers across the nation. Last summer, Los Angeles lawmakers banned fast-food chains from opening new outlets in South L.A., which has the city's highest concentration of fast-food restaurants and a 30 percent higher rate of obesity than the rest of Los Angeles County.[111] Just recently, the state of West Virginia – determined the unhealthiest state in the nation – passed legislation (almost unanimously) to ban drive-thru windows at fast-food restaurants.[112] And it's not only government that is paying attention. This past summer, Disney Corporation became one of the first corporations to publicly take a stand against this problem by banning junk-food ads aimed at kids on its television networks (including ABC, which Disney owns).[113]

What actually started the overweight revolution? Most likely, the roots of our current situation began in the 1970s when our national agricultural policy changed from paying farmers to grow only essential crops to encouraging them to grow as much food as they could. Newer fertilizers, pesticides, herbicides, irrigation techniques, and improvements in the capacity of farm equipment allowed farms to become much more productive. As huge amounts of food were grown, the prices plummeted, making it possible for an army of food producers to turn certain crops into gold – *processed foods.*

The number of calories available per person grew by 1000 calories a day, and we started overeating.[114] Since that time, as a nation we have obliterated our links to a past when people ate three meals a day, prepared food at home, and ate together as a family. Our mantra of everything in moderation has actually come to mean: eat anything that strikes your fancy, whenever you are awake, no matter the nutritional content, and with no regard for the consequences. We don't eat because we are hungry; we eat because we are craving something – whether a specific taste, relief from an uncomfortable feeling, or just because we are starved for nutrients. Yes, many of us (even though we are overweight) are starved for good nutrition; so we overeat the nutritionally deficient foods thinking this will satisfy us. But they never do. We don't buy food, we buy food products that were originally grown in nature but are now so highly processed that they have little relation to their natural origins. We buy things in cardboard boxes, plastic bags, plastic tubs, shrink-wrapped in cellophane on a Styrofoam™ plate – food-like items that last for months and in many cases even years on a shelf or in a freezer.

We build the most modern gourmet kitchens, but ironically most of us don't cook anymore; and when we do cook, we think

> We don't eat because we are hungry; we eat because we are craving something – whether a specific taste, relief from an uncomfortable feeling, or just because we are starved for nutrients.

that "nuking" a cheeseburger and fries or macaroni and cheese etc. in the microwave provides acceptable, health-promoting nutrition. Even more disturbing, we aren't convinced that vegetables and fruits should be consumed on a regular basis because they aren't comparatively convenient, unless of course they come in a can and are essentially devoid of any nutritional benefits. It's comical to some to consider that they might actually have to wash, peel, or cook a vegetable. Moreover, we have grown discontent with drinking water from public fountains (which is actually understandable on one level); however, we are instead demanding 16, 20 and 24 oz. highly sweetened beverages at our disposal 24 hours a day. And does anyone remember when it used to be considered improper, and a sign of poor manners, to eat in public? Now, we can't go outside without our favorite fructose-saturated sports drink, and we walk and drive around with our hands full of comestibles much of the time.

A study published in the journal *Appetite* found that the food industry works to "fundamentally change children's taste palates to increase their liking of highly processed and less nutritious foods."

Food preparation is routinely outsourced such that schools, hospitals and nursing homes rarely offer any fresh food. The meals purchased by schools for our children are prepared far away and far in advance of consumption. Schools are of particular concern, not only because our children receive around 50% of their daily calories on school grounds, but because schools are where our children learn. In this case, however, they are learning habits, including relying on vending machines for food, that will keep them obese and unhealthy for the rest of their lives.[115] Who is leading the charge to push industrial foods on kids rather than supplying what is healthy? Multinational corporations like ConAgra and Schwan. Making matters worse, our government representatives – so deeply and incestuously tied to political donations – have lost all common sense regarding the matter. It was just last November (2011) that Congress announced that frozen pizza qualified as a vegetable. Not only did they vote to rebuke new USDA guidelines for school lunches that would have increased the amount of fresh fruit and vegetables in school cafeterias, they declared that the sugar-laden tomato paste (on the nutritionally bankrupt white-flour frozen pizza dough) qualified as a vegetable.[116] Have we gone completely insane? Can you begin now to see the depth of this insanity, and how it is affecting our nation's health?

A recent article appearing in the *Huffington Post* noted the brilliance of the food industry – not only for creating these industrial foods, but for convincing us that processed food is *all* that children want, which may now be true.[117] Sadly, the industry spends billions of dollars on concocting highly addictive taste profiles that literally change children's palates. The author noted:

> "...eating sugary, salty and fatty food products adjusts taste preference to the point that simple, real foods taste bland and unappealing...While the food industry insists that it only advertises to children "to influence brand preference," a study published in the journal *Appetite* found that the food industry works to "fundamentally change children's taste palates to increase their liking of highly processed and less nutritious foods."

This is criminal in my opinion, and I feel saddened that we as a nation continue to fall prey to the deceit and trickery of corporations that care about one thing alone: *profits*. It is no secret that schools across America are financially stressed. Not only is it common for parents and teachers now to pay for school supplies, it has become necessary for school systems to entertain income from other sources – and the food industry is happy to "help." Traditional school lunch is no longer the only option. Now children are presented with a food court full of "competitive food" options like pizza, hot dogs, tater tots, French fries and sugary beverages including soda at breakfast and lunch. Schools view feeding children as a financial advantage, and necessary to their survival. They have placed vending machines in the hallways and teacher lounges so that packaged foods are available throughout the day. However, now that local and state governments are getting involved (albeit slowly) in the battle, appropriate changes are occurring – and working. A report in the *New York Times Health & Science* section in May of this year spoke about California's success in the fight against obesity in our youth.[118] Just five years after they began cracking down on junk food in school cafeterias, it was stated that high school students there consume fewer calories (approximately 160 calories per student per day) and less fat and sugar at school than students in other states. Researchers believe that California's wholesale shift is helping: they have not only eliminated sweets and candy bars; they have banned soda, and legislated nutritional guidelines for so called "competitive foods."

The problem in schools is magnified by the dismantling of physical education programs over the past 20 years. According to recent research conducted by a University of Georgia professor and published in the *Journal of Teaching in Physical Education*, schools in all 50 states are uniformly failing at implementing state mandates for school-based physical education.[119,120] The results found only six states mandate the appropriate guidelines – 150 minutes each week – for elementary school physical education, which boils down to only 30 minutes a day. Moreover, only two states mandate the appropriate amount for middle schools, and none at the high school level – 225 minutes weekly for both. He

Schools in all 50 states are uniformly failing at implementing state mandates for school-based physical education.

– Journal of Teaching in Physical Education

cites the lack of national mandates and federal judicial support on state mandates coupled with budgetary challenges as the primary reasons for state noncompliance. It doesn't help that "an estimated 40 percent of U.S. school districts either have eliminated recess or are considering eliminating it," according to an article published by the PTA.[121] Another article published recently in *the Atlantic* said: "Even more important, as play and recess have declined over the past half-century, anxiety, depression, suicide, feelings of helplessness and narcissism have increased, suggesting a connection between play and children's long-term mental health."[122] Findings by the CDC are similar; according to a 2010 report: "...studies found one or more positive associations between recess and indicators of cognitive skills, attitudes, and academic behavior."[123]

Corporations also continue to add to the problem *outside* of schools by offering cleverly disguised "reward" programs for ice cream and other junk foods in partnership with organizations and initiatives focused on, of all things, child safety! Both McDonalds and Dairy Queen are regular participants in a program that advocates helmet use during bicycling, where local, on-duty police officers distribute coupons to obedient children. Having, of all people, police officers – natural role models who enjoy an extremely high social rank and authority in the minds of youngsters – distribute these coupons has a tremendous psychological impact, and fiscal one too. After all, what child wouldn't follow through on an offer extended by a police officer, and continue to frequent these fast food outlets throughout life because a police officer encouraged them to at a very young age? What an incredibly creative, insidious and cost-effective way (using government services funded by tax-payers) for these corporations to pedal their unhealthy fare to budding lifelong customers.

Bombarded by ceaseless advertising for the interest of increasing corporate profits by way of lifelong patients, as in the case of arthritis, we have become a nation out of control. The food industry spends $1.6 billion a year in predatory food advertising to our children alone.[124] There is relentless peer pressure to consume these industrial foods and beverages, and the media and our health professionals act as if all food items are the same: "there are no bad foods," we are often told. So you won't ever hear what's wrong with energy drinks, bagels, or egg, sausage and cheese sandwiches on white bread.

Because obesity is both a cause *and* result of arthritis, we are obliged – as a nation engaged in a full-fledged health crisis – to view the type of foods being promoted and pushed on our children early in their life, and the loss and lack of physical exercise as the dangerous and deadly combination that it is. Until we address the root cause – a cultural lifestyle shift to consuming significantly increased and nutritionally void calories with little to no expenditure of energy – we will remain absorbed in a risk of monumental proportions as opposed to taking real action for real change.

But without the needed action, we simply adjust. As long as the meals are full of processed fats, salt and sugars, and satisfy some inner craving, we don't complain. We don't worry when we start putting on weight and develop joint pain because everyone else is putting on weight too. We don't even seem to worry when our health deteriorates – when not only we but our children have high blood pressure and diabetes. And we are more worried about preventing a decline in self-esteem because of our overweight appearance and our need to appear attractive than we are about making changes to restore our health. Instead, we listen to those industry spokespeople who argue that you can be fat and healthy too. Just take a pill.

As we have seen, it's not only the corporations that we know – like McDonalds and Dairy Queen – behind the advertising and media front, but the meat and dairy farmers and manufacturers, processed food manufacturers (including chemical and flavoring companies), the pharmaceutical and medical industries, and our government. We simply don't recognize that these factions and the media that they own are complicit in putting us exactly where they want us. We have been conditioned like Pavlovian dogs, and don't stop to question why we have arthritis. We also are not questioning what and how much are we eating, and why our consumption is making us sick, and even killing us.

The more our bodies break down, the more we become beholden to Big Pharma as well as the medical and surgical establishment to keep us alive (but not healthy) with medications for these chiefly lifestyle diseases. We are persuaded by the constant reinforcement of the propaganda machine to buy food items that we don't need: subliminal advertising creates desire. There are few rules for advertising claims and no standards: you can make virtually any declaration about a processed food with no proof, as long as the nutritional label on the reverse of the package provides certain required information – albeit in small print – and the few rules of the game are adhered to. An example of the ludicrousness in food advertising is a fat-free spray-on oil where the only ingredient is 100% fat! Other processed "fat-free" foods are so laden with sugar and chemicals that they have been identified by most nutritionists as a serious health risk.

Regrettably, it's not just products in cardboard boxes that we need to be wary of. Despite overwhelming dissent from consumers and scientists, the FDA declared in 2008 that meat and dairy companies do not need to inform consumers when the product is a result of cloning. While, the FDA has issued three reports confirming the safety of these products, they remain questionable by consumers and scientists alike; and, as reported in *Newsweek Magazine*, there is some evidence that cloned animals show a higher propensity for developmental problems.[125] Biologists – notoriously and rightly skeptical of such simplistic notions that copying DNA from a prize cow will result in a prized cow – are particular flummoxed by proponents' overly enthusiastic assessments. And while some scientific tests may say that cloned meat has the same technical composition as non-cloned meat, none are conducting studies on differences in how the meat is handled by the human body. Unfortunately, this is just another example of scientific study in action – with the American public as the primary test subject. As a sufferer of arthritis, you will want to do all you can to avoid industrialized foods including cloned and genetically engineered foods and eat as much organic plant-based food as possible, which protects you from the injurious effects of "foods" created by an overzealous scientific and food industry community.

With limited labeling legislation and little or no guidance about what constitutes a healthy food, parents are frequently too overwhelmed with their work and their children's school and social activities to plan and prepare nutritious meals. The truth is that most Americans can and do eat whatever and whenever they want, seemingly under the impression or belief that nearly all foods lead to good health – even though there is evidence to the contrary right in front of our eyes if we look. Yet it doesn't persuade us to question the food or advertising industries, the medical establishment, or our legislators, including our food regulatory agency the FDA. Perhaps what is of most concern here is that unless we are very old, chances are that most of us never really learned the basics of healthy eating, and probably won't.

The Difficulty of Improving Our Toxic Food Landscape

Many of you may remember the beef industry's response to Oprah Winfrey in 1996 when she expressed her opinion on her popular television show about the dangers of eating beef.

Trampling on the First Amendment (the right to freedom of speech), the beef industry took her to court. How was it that they were able to sue Oprah? Because in 1995, the state of Texas passed legislation making it illegal to disparage perishable food products. In the end, after a long and drawn-out battle over six years, Oprah triumphed – but only because of her vast financial reserves, which

> I f you suffer from arthritis, you are also likely suffering from the influence of these powerful players, as well as a medical system that by nature of its focus to eradicate symptoms can only fail you.

allowed her to mount an adequate defense.[126] Did she say anything that was inaccurate or untrue about the dangers of beef? No, but the truth doesn't count for much in this game. The evidence is that as individuals we are largely powerless to fight the influence of the food industry, supported by unethical legislators, to break the stranglehold it has on what is available to us as food in America.

Indeed we are dealing with a monstrous, intricately woven system of collusion. In 2007, a few intrepid researchers set out to do a study on the how funding sources affect the nutritional information that is published in scientific articles. They looked at funding sources of four types of scientific studies dealing with soft drinks, juice, and milk published between 1999 and 2003. What they found was that scientific articles about these particular beverages funded by industry were four to eight times more likely to be favorable to the financial interests of the sponsors. Furthermore, none of the interventional studies supported by the beverage industry, which investigated likelihood of certain responses to consumption of certain beverages, such as gaining weight or developing diabetes, had unfavorable conclusions.[127]

Beginning in 2009, the Interagency Working Group (IWG) was assembled to examine the issue of junk food marketing to children and to develop voluntary guidelines restricting this practice in response to the current and growing obesity epidemic. The group determined that their recommendations should support two basic goals: first, that foods marketed to children should provide nutrients from healthy food groups, such as fruits, vegetables, and whole grains; and second, that foods marketed to children should be made with minimal amounts of unhealthy ingredients including saturated fat, trans-fats, sugar, and sodium.[128]

Initially, the IWG seemed to have broad based bipartisan support, and they released their proposed guidelines in April 2011. While comments from consumers and public health groups strongly supported the proposed guidelines, the food industry put pressure on legislators through monetary contributions and lobbying from front groups falsely claiming to represent consumers. An eventual tsunami of outrage poured forth toward the IWG from both the Republican and Democratic legislators compensated by the food industry. They expressed outrage that the IWG intended to discriminate against an industry that "has made extensive voluntary strides" to reduce advertising to children. In the end, food industry money turned the tide. Not only was the plan scrapped, but the IWG was prohibited from working on the guidelines without complying with certain stringent requirements in the omnibus spending bill passed in December 2011.[129]

The requirements, which would have taken many years' worth of analysis and reports, effectively quashed the effort to limit junk food marketing to children. The seemingly high price of the reported $37 million spent by the food industry to oppose the IWG recommendations was clearly well worth the price.[130]

The relentless advertising of unhealthy food products (including those portended to be healthy) to children and adults continues because selling products that are a cause of obesity and chronic poor health is, in fact, a goldmine for the multinational corporations that manufacture them, and for the medical system that is assigned to fix the problems they create. If you suffer from arthritis, you are also likely suffering from the influence of these powerful players, as well as a medical system that by nature of its focus to eradicate symptoms can only fail you.

Our only defense is an individual one: not only must we arm ourselves with information the industry does not want us to have, but we must take actions like those outlined in this book that are in alignment with creating a healthy existence free from disease-causing factors. Equally important is sharing this information, as well as the knowledge you gain by making healthier choices, with others. Together, we can make strides.

In spite of the difficulty of achieving success over our seemingly intractable system, it may be worthy of our attempt as citizens to involve ourselves in ways that are appropriate to our circumstances, including "voting with our dollars." To start, consider purchasing only organic foods, and from local farmers. This is a wonderful way of supporting the change that you wish to see. Also, get involved in the legislative process – even on a local basis. Ask the difficult questions, and educate others about alternatives. There are numerous individuals who through class-action law suits have championed over corporations in defective product lawsuits.

The Standard American Diet (SAD)

So what is specifically wrong with the American way of eating? Plenty! We need certain nutrients to survive. Our daily intake of food must contain protein, starch, fat, vegetables and fruit in enough quantity to support good health without causing the deposition of excess fat. Because of its reliance on packaged, processed food the Standard American Diet contains far too much fat, refined carbohydrate, sugar, salt and artificial ingredients – and it's killing us. Heart disease, diabetes, cancer, Alzheimer's and other fatal diseases are on the increase, with no signs of stopping.

In general, the majority of the modern medical community remains ignorant of the critical role of a whole-foods diet in the creation and maintenance of optimal health. Physicians in training are required to take few courses on nutrition. Once they are in practice, they are barraged by pharmaceutical company reps with convincing messages of powerful drugs claimed to alleviate *symptoms*, which is "good enough" right now – in the sense that you aren't actually dying. My colleague Dr. Dillard says it this way: "Medical doctors spend most of their education identifying and treating things that are going to kill us *quickly* as opposed to the things that are killing us slowly. It simply would be considered "bad form" for a doctor to miss something so obviously life threatening."

There is no comparison in nutritional value of a piece of chicken which has no antioxidants or phytochemicals and a piece of broccoli, which has thousands!

But what is the actual *cause* of physical disease? How do we create and maintain health? And, why are we getting sick in record numbers? In truth, without a regular supply of vitamins, minerals, phytochemicals (chemicals in plants having biological significance but are not established as essential nutrients), and other micronutrients, we simply cannot be healthy. The Standard American Diet (SAD) is dehydrating, acid-producing (rather than alkalizing) and suppresses the immune system. It is promoting obesity and chronic disease at alarming rates. Americans currently eat:

- 2.5% whole grains
- 10% unrefined plant foods: vegetables (including deep-fried white potato as in French fries, ironically the most-consumed "vegetable" in the US), fruit, beans, nuts and seeds
- 25.5% meat, eggs, dairy, fish
- 62% processed food: oil, sweets, refined grains[131]

In general our diet consists of incredibly tasty, addictive, calorie-dense food items that contain few or no nutrients. These foods tend to be easy to chew and come in quantities that are easy to *over*indulge in – like a bag of potato chips, a bucket of wings, a plate of nachos. We also drink our calories: since 1977, the consumption of sugar-sweetened beverages has increased by at least 135%![132]

While we may not be starving in one sense of the word, the cells in our bodies *are* starving – for nutrients (defined as a substance that provides nourishment essential for growth and the maintenance of life). Our immune function is supported by and thrives on the consumption of antioxidants and phytochemicals found in unrefined plant foods, and it is weakened and damaged by a diet high in processed foods. Most Americans are dramatically deficient in plant phytochemicals due to our longstanding practice of consuming a diet of processed foods. Neither processed foods nor animal products, which make up the bulk of the Standard American Diet, contain a significant amount of antioxidants or phytochemicals, the absence of which leads to chronic nutritional deficiencies and disease. There is no comparison in nutritional value of a piece of chicken which has no antioxidants or phytochemicals and a piece of broccoli, which has thousands!

Furthermore, an inadequate diet starting in childhood can create cellular damage leading to serious illnesses – besides obesity – in adulthood, which may be impossible to correct. Without a diet rich in antioxidants and phytochemicals, we are subject to oxidative stress and cellular damage from free radicals, which leads to premature aging, degenerative diseases, infection, and cancer.

Another significant problem linked to the Standard American Diet is that it is fast, as in "fast food" – meaning we eat on the run, often while we are doing other things and without attention to satiation. Closely tied to this is the newly developed cultural behavior of "grazing," which has become our primary approach to food consumption. Without defined meal times and limitations on the number of meals in a day, or the amount and quality of food eaten, there is no way Americans could be anything but overweight. We cling to the illusion that we are eating when we are hungry and stopping when we are full, but this hasn't been the case for the average American for the past 30 years. Otherwise, we wouldn't be experiencing our current obesity crisis. Most Americans no longer recognize hunger because they so rarely experience it. Full now means overcapacity, almost to the point of vomiting. Our stomachs are flexible and have a tremendous ability to stretch without bursting. Unfortunately, many abuse this on a daily basis and are suffering the consequences as a result.

> "**S**ince 1977, the consumption of sugar-sweetened beverages has increased by at least 135%"

Food Addiction

Little discussed in the popular press – and vehemently denied by the purveyors of junk food – is the fact that our standard diet is composed of many processed foods which are, in fact, addictive. Scientists in all the major food companies work hard to find the right combination of flavors (mostly artificial) to make processed food irresistible and, I will say this again...*addictive.* These foods change our palates and our body chemistry so that we want more and more of them. Whether the end result is sweet or salty, virtually all processed foods have a combination of fat, sugar, and salt, so that we become entrained to strong *and* certain tastes: ice cream, pizza, cookies, cupcakes, doughnuts, French fries, macaroni and cheese, Twinkies, etc. No one runs to the store at one o'clock in the morning for a pint of broccoli, but how many people believe they simply have to satisfy food cravings regardless of the hour? A 2009 study by Brownell and Gearhardt at Yale University examined the similarity of food addiction and substance abuse. They found that out of 350 Yale undergraduates, 11% reported:

- loss of control when eating,
- persistent desire or effort to cut back on intake, and
- excessive food consumption despite deleterious consequences.

They even created the Yale Food Addiction Scale with the intention to study this phenomenon in wider groups.[133]

A 2001 study entitled "Brain Dopamine and Obesity" by G. Wang and Nora Volkow, of the Brookhaven National Laboratory, showed that science supports the concept that the brain is taken over by certain foods, just like with particular drugs.[134] This groundbreaking research showed that not only can people become addicted to highly processed foods, but that obese people have brain MRI scans which resemble those of drug addicts rather than non-addicted people. Dopamine is a neurotransmitter (a chemical released by nerve cells to send signals to other nerve cells) made in the brain that causes a feeling of well-being. Not only does the body tend to seek out those things that raise the level of dopamine, but if there aren't many receptors in an individual's brain, then more of a substance or activity to generate that pleasurable feeling is needed. Low levels of dopamine D2 receptors have been demonstrated in the brains of people addicted to cocaine, opiates, and alcohol. Dr. Volkow's study showed that there is likewise a low level of D2 receptors in obese people and that the amount of these receptors is inversely correlated with BMI: the heavier the person, the fewer D2 receptors present in the brain. Furthermore, the lack of D2 receptors in obese individuals may perpetuate pathological eating behavior. According to Dr. Volkow, certain foods can commandeer the brain in ways that resemble addictions to cocaine, nicotine and other drugs. "The data is so overwhelming the field has to accept it...We are finding tremendous overlap between drugs in the brain and food in the brain."[135]

Obese people have significantly fewer dopamine receptors in a part of the brain called the striatum. With fewer receptors, obese people need to eat far more than a normal-weight person to experience the same 'high'.[136] Also, after a meal of highly processed addictive food, once the high wears off, withdrawal is so unpleasant that people want to eat more to make themselves feel better. This makes becoming overweight inevitable. If we stop digesting food, even for a short time, our bodies begin to experience symptoms of detoxification or withdrawal from our unhealthful diet. To counter this, we keep our digestive track overfed to lessen the discomfort of this stressful style of diet.[137]

It would be extremely rare to find someone addicted to a food grown in nature – such as broccoli or apples – to the point that they would eat it to excess. But processed foods are created using scientific research that has proven what flavors or substances cause craving in order to sell as much product as possible. Studies have shown that a combination of sugar, fat, and salt is irresistible to a large number of people, so these three appear in combination in the vast majority of processed foods: the end result is overeating.

Reducing overall calories, adopting a healthy diet, avoiding addictive (processed) foods, and starting a regular exercise program can increase dopamine receptors, which would eventually allow a person to feel well more consistently, and have a better chance at achieving and maintaining a normal weight.

The good news is that the loss of dopamine receptors does not appear to be irreversible. Evidence shows the brain's ability to produce dopamine can be repaired. Pharmacological studies indicate that enhanced dopamine activity is associated with reduced food intake. The key, then, to overcoming food addiction begins with a complete change in diet, which would facilitate weight loss.[138] Reducing overall calories, adopting a healthy diet, avoiding addictive (processed) foods, and starting a regular exercise program can increase dopamine receptors, which would eventually allow a person to feel well more consistently, and have a better chance at achieving and maintaining a normal weight. Longer, moderate intensity exercise is best for elevating dopamine, as well as other pertinent mood neurotransmitters such as serotonin and endorphins. Besides the physiological benefits of increased energy, strength and relaxation (post-exercise), the psychological benefits of exercise (and the related increase in dopamine levels) are vast and crucial for people with debilitating diseases such as arthritis. When we have a disease, especially one with pain, it can be challenging to be focused on positive thoughts and actions; exercise is excellent for this. In addition to reducing anxiety and stress, regular exercise improves self-esteem, body image, confidence, brain function and mood, as well as an overall improvement in feelings of well-being. (Read more about exercise in Section III of this book.)

Perhaps even more so than dietary therapy, health professionals agree on the importance of exercise. A scientific statement from the *Council on Clinical Cardiology* and the *Council on Nutrition, Physical Activity, and Metabolism* endorsed and published by the *American Heart Association* stated: "The importance of physical activity for health and the use of exercise training in managing selected disease states should be incorporated into the education of physicians and other medical professionals. A physical activity history is an important component of the health history, and healthcare providers should include the patient's habitual physical activity as part of the medical record. Healthcare providers should identify for patients the importance of physical activity as primary or adjunctive therapy for such medical conditions as hypertension, hypertriglyceridemia, glucose intolerance, and obesity."[139] The findings are unanimous across the board: the *National Parkinson Foundation* says "we know that people who exercise intensely, for example by doing things like running or riding a bicycle, have fewer changes in their brains caused by aging;" and according to a study done by a group of scientists in 1995, "rheumatoid arthritis patients die 10 to 15 years earlier than non-afflicted individuals. But, the research shows a predictably higher mortality rate in RA patients who are inactive." [140]

The High Cost of Cheap Food

On the whole, we are spending less on food than ever before while, at the same time, we are spending more on health care. Value meals are now the cornerstone of the main fast food establishments. At McDonalds, Burger King *and* Taco Bell you can get a meal for $1.00, and a bag of potato chips in a low-income neighborhood bodega costs only $0.25.

What could possibly propel these lower than realistic food costs? In part, our farm policy is driving farmers to overproduce crops that we are already overeating, namely corn and soy. Fast food giants, who can dictate crop production, also have tremendous buying power – because of the quantities of food they purchase they pay far less for the same product than most. This is what allows them to give away meals for ridiculously low prices; what they don't make up on volume from increased market share they make up in extra product sales. The point is that we're getting a better deal on processed foods than if we were paying the real cost of the meal, but we are mortgaging our long term health and the country's economy in the process. Most farmers no longer view what they grow as food but as a commodity that will become livestock feed or high fructose corn syrup for soft drinks or calorie-laden snacks. How did we ever get to this point – so far away from natural foods, and humans caring far more about their own welfare than that of their fellow citizens? The 15 billion dollars a year we spend to grow corn and soybeans, which are then turned into processed foods, actually costs us hundreds of billions of dollars annually to treat obesity-related illnesses.[141]

The cost of fruit and vegetables has risen by 117% since the 1980s while the cost of soft drinks has gone up by only 20%. Part of the reason for this is that we don't grow enough fruits and vegetables in this country to meet our own dietary recommendations. As unbelievable and alarming a fact as this is, less than 3% of U.S. farmland is planted with fruits and vegetables.[142] Even more confounding is that the economic incentives of globalization force us to accept foreign-grown produce, even in areas where these crops are grown in our own country – like grapes being imported from Chile for use in California. If the farm subsidy were eliminated, for example, it could become more cost effective for farmers to grow fruits and vegetables.

Stress

As time goes on, I believe that already mounting evidence about the deleterious effects of stress and its relationship to illness will expand significantly. In fact, my colleague Jill R. Baron, M.D., Integrative Medicine Physician and Weight-loss Specialist believes that most illness begins in the mind, and in the brain, with stress. She says, "When you have stress, your body *and* your cells do not function optimally. This is especially the case with chronic stress." This statement has support from many others, and some leaders in this field of study. I first interviewed Dr. Hans Selye, the famous Hungarian endocrinologist internationally acknowledged as "the father of the stress field," in 1972. Selye, who was nominated for the Nobel Prize as many as 10 times, coined the term "distress"

There are thousands of studies in peer-reviewed literature on psychoneuroimmunology, showing that what you think, you become.

therapy, suggesting that it is not stress per se, but what he called "adverse stress" that causes problems. After all, when you are doing something that makes you happy, that creates a positive stress. Going to the theater, a baseball game or engaging in a sport, for example, is constructive. On the other hand, Selye emphasized that every time you think a negative thought, you create a negative biochemistry. Cortisol, epinephrine, norepinephrine, catecholamines, and an elevation in blood sugar all follow distress. So low level anxiety and worry, a sense of foreboding (the type of gloom and doom that is so common today), even a person fearing their own mortality as they age, generally starting at age 40 and increasing with every decade beyond (meaning they have an increased awareness of their expiration date), are all examples of the chronic low-level stressors that can make us feel unsettled in life.

Today, in particular, you can add in the fear of financial insecurity, which is so prevalent now with over 100 million Americans at the poverty level, and over 15 million senior citizens not having enough money to pay their bills. Moreover, financial stress frequently causes relationship stress, which manifests as ongoing arguments. Then, the entire fabric of a relationship can become unraveled. Nothing in America is perfectly stable today if you are the average person; only the rich and powerful know where their next meal is coming from. There is also uncertainty about where we live: 16 states are now in permanent drought, and quality of life there has been compromised. This is not to mention permanent damage to the areas in our country affected by hurricanes, and other disasters – natural or manmade. Daily concerns have exacerbated the production of stress hormones in many Americans. These silent hormones create inflammatory biochemicals and increase oxidative stress.

You can see the effects of stress by looking at the physical signs of aging (like greying hair) in a president after just four years in office. The damage occurs in the inner cells and translates to changes in the outer (cells that we can see). And for so many people, stress can contribute to inflammation in musculature and joints, causing pain and arthritis. This is why in every meeting of our anti-arthritis support group we emphasize positive thinking to creating positive biochemistry. There are thousands of studies in peer-reviewed literature on psychoneuroimmunology, showing that what you think, you become. Think a stressful, angry, negative, or foreboding thought, and you have just turned on the pro-inflammatory biochemistry. Positive spiritual thoughts turn on the healing biochemistry.

As a country, there is no doubt that we continue to underestimate the role of stress in our health crises, and we will continue to pay the price until its causes are addressed. According to the *National Health Interview Survey*, 75% of the general population experiences at least "some stress" every two weeks.[143] Additionally, worker's compensation claims for "mental stress" in California rose 200-700% in the 1980s (whereas all other causes remained stable or declined.) The National Institute of Mental Health says an estimated 26.2 percent of Americans ages 18 and older – about one in four adults – suffer from a diagnosable mental disorder in a given year.[144] When combined with 2004 U.S. Census information, this figure translates to 57.7 million people, and nearly half (45 percent) of those with any diagnosable mental disorder meet criteria for two or more mental disorders.[145]

The frightening thing about stress is that it not only causes disease, it causes us to take actions – like drink, smoke and overeat – that create further disease and stress. Unfortunately, as a culture we have not yet developed, on the whole, a healthy approach to managing stress. While our awareness is increasing, and we are engaging more in activities like yoga, meditation, and regular exercise, the majority of us are still using tranquilizers, antidepressants, and antianxiety medications to handle our stress, as they account for one fourth of all prescriptions written in the U.S. each year.[146] We also use food, alcohol, work, violence and sex (to name a few) in excess because we have not learned how to manage our fears and the chaos created by our minds with the changing tides in life.

As you will see later in the book, recovery from chronic illness such as arthritis requires the cultivation of awareness – not only of what is happening in our body, but of what is happening in our mind that is either helping or harming us in our quest for health. If you have any doubt about the power of your mind, consider eliminating your favorite unhealthy food – the one that you "cannot live without" – for just one week. Whether coffee (caffeine), tobacco, sugar, dairy or alcohol, you will quickly realize how difficult this can be – not just physically, but mentally and emotionally. The mind is extremely powerful, more so than you can imagine, and it will prevent you from doing what you know is best for your body if you cannot see how it creates endless reasons and excuses to meet the discomforts of life head on. After you get through the first week or few weeks of eliminating that toxic food, however, you inevitably feel better. You have more energy, mental clarity and an overall feeling of increased vitality.

Simple acts like breathing consciously and deeply throughout the day, being mindful when we are eating, having a spiritual practice, forming loving bonds with people, cultivating a realistic and proper perspective about life, and taking time for rest, relaxation, enjoyment, and play are all critical factors for health. There is no way that we can be truly healthy without managing our stress in healthful ways. In Section III of this book, we give you a list of proven techniques for reducing your stress.

- 4 -

Addressing Diseases of Inflammation

When addressing any *dis*-ease, it is crucial for us to focus our attention on repairing the *causes* of the disease, rather than just the symptoms, otherwise the disease will remain. While treating the symptoms may cause their cessation, it is only temporary. They will return so long as the underlying factors are not addressed.

Entering the System

When it comes to most diseases, including arthritis, there are essentially two ways of entering treatment – through conventional or natural medicine. While it is possible to combine these approaches, the priorities and methods associated with the treatment protocols of each vary greatly. I encourage as many people as possible to enter the system through a naturopathic or acupuncture physician, especially if prevention is your key concern. As I covered in earlier chapters, conventional methodologies do not actually treat the root cause of arthritis and, therefore, cannot offer any possibility of prevention or reversal. Natural treatments can offer this because they address the underlying imbalances that cause tissue degeneration. When you enter the system from the natural side, you have a much better chance of handling your illness thoroughly and permanently while creating improved health in the long run. Perhaps the most valuable thing to keep in mind on your journey with arthritis is the importance of embracing natural methodologies *as soon as possible*. If you wait too long, you run the risk of not being able to reverse the disease to a point where you regain enough functionality to enjoy life. I encourage you to get all the support that you need to get started now; the recommendations within this book work, and they will have a positive impact on your overall health and well-being extremely quickly. The power is yours, as is the ability, and you will be pleasantly surprised with the results.

Conventional methodologies do not actually treat the root cause of arthritis and, therefore, cannot offer any possibility of prevention or reversal.

The Route of Conventional Treatment

People who begin to experience stiffness or discomfort in their knees and hips, or a loss of range of motion, commonly see a physician for advice. In many cases, x-rays are taken to evaluate joint degeneration, and signs of a problem are usually found. This typically leads to a rapid surge of treatments even prior to the real cause of the problem being identified. My colleague Daniel Nuchovich, M.D. says "Many doctors rush in with colorful pills and recommendations for surgery before the *cause* is actually determined; this practice is a disservice to anyone with arthritis."

The issue with using x-rays or MRIs to diagnose arthritis is that studies show a very poor correlation between radiographic evidence of joint changes and loss of function. Pain specialist Dr. Dillard shared with me that the vast majority of his patients who exhibit arthritis on radiographic images are actually pain free. The research demonstrates that many people with degenerative joint disease on x-rays do not suffer from any disability, and likewise many who complain of problems have normal radiographs, but this is rarely explained to the patient.[147] Instead, radiographic "proof" of joint disease usually leads to immediate prescriptions for anti-inflammatory drugs, and recommendations for possible surgical interventions depending on the level of pain. The dreaded pronouncement of "bone on bone," of course, sends you right to the surgery suite. One prescription medication is generally not the end, others are soon added. Some medications may agree with you while others may not, and there is typically a trial and error process. Worse is that you may be on other medications for another disease, such as diabetes, atherosclerosis, etc. In this event, the introduction of an additional pharmaceutical creates a new biochemical dynamic that could result in the need of yet another drug to address the side effects from the initial one.

Meanwhile, unless steps are being taken to institute dietary and exercise therapy, the tissues continue to degenerate, and the arthritis advances. The conventional route is a frightening and dangerous prospect that leads to an almost certain demise, including becoming an arthritis patient for life. Because we hear so much about arthritis, and are bombarded with advertisements for arthritis medications and surgical centers, we assume that it is not a question of *if* but *when* we will become an arthritis sufferer. We now know that it doesn't have to be this way; living a healthy, balanced life and making natural health protocols a priority go a long way in preventing and eradicating arthritis.

The Route of Natural Treatment

While commonly mislabeled as "alternative" therapies, natural therapies have indeed existed for many thousands of years – far longer than our modern medical technologies. In today's medical community, you will hear these therapies called "complementary," for the reason that they serve as a complement to modern applications. Both of these names point to an incorrect belief that modern Western medicine is the "best" and "most important" form of medicine, and should be the primary form for the diseases that ail us. This couldn't be farther from the truth. In fact, eating natural foods, utilizing natural therapies, and living as naturally as possible, free from toxic influences, are the *only* ways to actually "cure" the lifestyle diseases that plague most Americans at this time.

> "Health is the proper relationship between microcosm, which is man, and the macrocosm, which is the universe. Disease is a disruption of this relationship."
>
> – *Dr. Yeshe Donden,*
> *Doctor of Tibetan Medicine and former*
> *physician to His Holiness the Dalai Lama*

Natural therapies such as acupuncture, massage, and dietary therapy are customs and techniques deeply rooted in ancient history. Many reports indicate they are at least 4,000 years old, and some say that massage has been around since the beginning of modern civilization. Regardless of the time they have been in place, the main thing is that they be recognized by *everyone* in our society as essential for a healthy, long, pain-free life. With this recognition, these therapies can assume their rightful place in our currently ailing healthcare system.

The terms "integrative health" and "integrative therapies" are two that I would suggest are more appropriate for evolving a healthcare system with true power and integrity – one that recognizes the obvious limitations of modern medicine but recognizes and advocates the tremendous value of natural medicine. A system like this would promote a healthier society overall and would also be sustainable for *humanity*, rather than just self-interested corporations and systems. We are talking about the lives of human beings here, and until we collectively see how far we have strayed from nature, and how much it is harming us, we will not change our situation. Obviously, there are modern inventions that have proven invaluable in humanity's quest for an optimally healthful life; however, without a tried and true effort to understand all the factors involved in our increasingly deteriorating state, we will remain tied to modern medicine's harmful remedies and incomplete protocols of symptomatic relief, and miss the bigger opportunity.

Speaking of which, when embarking upon an arthritis treatment program through a natural practitioner such as a Naturopathic physician, a Doctor of Acupuncture, a Doctor of Osteopathy, or Chiropractor there is one thing that is consistently the same across the board. Nearly all of these practitioners begin their analysis and eventual treatment of your illness with a comprehensive health and nutritional profile, including appropriate testing. All of these medical professionals are interested in treating the "whole" person, not just one area of the body. In addition to understanding your prior medical treatment history, they will ask you about critical factors such as how much you sleep, what supplements you take, how much exercise you get, how happy you are at your job, and the primary stressors in your life. The training for all of these professions is deeply rooted in the foundational concept that a person's illness cannot be separate from the person itself, and that illness almost always results from mental, emotional, spiritual *and* physical *dis*ease. In fact, Dr. Yeshe Donden, world-renowned Doctor of Tibetan Medicine and former physician to His Holiness the Dalai Lama has said: "Health is the proper relationship between microcosm, which is man, and the macrocosm, which is the universe. Disease is a disruption of this relationship."

Indeed, this is the belief held by natural medicine practitioners. My colleague Chinese Medicine Doctor of Acupuncture Peter Bongiorno, N.D., L.Ac. says "We need to think about our spirit in the treatment of arthritis and pain. When we are doing the things we love, following our passion, and our lives are relatively balanced and not too stressful, we are creating a healthy environment for our body. When we are not following the path that we believe we should, it causes a lot of internal stress. In Chinese Medicine, the heart spirit affects all the other organ systems and stops things from working properly, and this can create issues later on that we are pre-disposed to, like arthritis." Dr. Bongiorno continued: "I always ask people if they are doing the things that they love, if their relationships are healthy, and if not, what steps can be taken to change those situations. If people are not following their passions at work, I ask them how they can get involved in the things that they are passionate about outside of work. I believe – and have seen from my experience – that the body tells us when our spirit isn't in alignment with how we are living; and when we take steps to do what makes our heart happy, our body responds." [148]

This is a far different intake approach than on the allopathic side, which is mainly concerned with previous illnesses, surgeries and current medications. Can you see the difference already? A survey of doctors by *Consumer Reports* (reported in *Newsweek Magazine*) said that 70 percent of doctors reported that the bond with their patients has eroded since they began practicing medicine.[149] At the heart of the problem, say doctors, is the managed-care revolution of the 1980s and '90s, which resulted in lower reimbursements to doctors, making it necessary for them to slash the amount of time spent with patients in order to see more patients in a day (and make the same amount of money). Because doctors are typically paid for the number of procedures as well as number of patients they see – *and not for the time that they spend* – there is a very real incentive for them to spend less time. Findings have estimated that on average, patients can expect to spend no more than 10 to 16 minutes with their doctor, with an average around 7 minutes![150,151] In contrast, most naturopathic physicians spend anywhere from one to two hours (6-12 times the amount of time spent with an allopathic physician) on the initial visit, and one-half hour each on return visits. [152] The longer visits are not only related to more in-depth questioning on the doctor's part but include educating a patient about the causes of disease *and* wellness.

What actually can be learned and determined about a person and their disease in 7-15 minutes? If the treatment of your illness – and, therefore, your quality of life – depends on multiple factors regarding many areas of your life, wouldn't you feel more comfortable with a health professional that is schooled to *look for* and *assess* the causes of *dis*-ease, and then address them in the treatment program? I cannot stress the value of working with health practitioners who will listen to you, educate you about what is happening in your body, and discuss your options with you. I've worked with numerous natural practitioners in my years as a pioneer in nutritional education, and every one of them has told me this: You have to truly want to be well in order to be well because it takes education and consistent application. This reminds me of something that John Knowles, Former President of the Rockefeller Foundation, said: "The next major advance in the health of the American people will be determined by what the individual is willing to do for himself."

In terms of education, many natural doctors and practitioners have a broad understanding of exercise and plant-based nutrition their value in maintaining health. Most take training in the use

Findings have estimated that on average, patients can expect to spend no more than 10 to 16 minutes with their doctor, with an average around 7 minutes!

of nutritional supplements and create alliances with companies that offer high-quality products. Several give classes and talks in the community about staying healthy. If they do not already have other natural practitioners on staff, such as massage therapists and nutritionists (which often they do), to assist their patients, they will make appropriate referrals to colleagues with other areas of expertise, as well as offer suggestions on books and other resources.

In terms of the treatment program, natural doctors will typically develop a protocol (including benchmark goals for improvement) *after* the initial visit. They will discuss the protocol and suggest actions that you can take to improve your condition at a follow-up visit. As mentioned before, blood tests and other clinical testing may be ordered to assess your overall condition. One of the first things that many naturopaths will do in addressing arthritis is to make certain that your vitamin and mineral levels are strong and balanced. Low levels of nutrients are a factor in inflammation and, therefore, arthritic conditions, so they must be dealt with as a first course of action. If you aren't already on a multivitamin and multi-mineral supplement, chances are this will be recommended, along with the inclusion of other key supplements like omega-3s (from algae or fish oil), glucosamine/chondroitin, and key antioxidants. (See Section II & III of this book for a more in-depth explanation of supplements.)

There is much more interest and care, overall, in how your *life* is improving with the protocol, and not just your arthritis symptoms. Natural practitioners will recommend testing at benchmark periods to improve the effectiveness of their treatments, and will make referrals to and work with conventional medical doctors if necessary. In general, natural practitioners are oriented toward restoring your wellness, which means stopping the progression of arthritis – and even reversing it. Their aim is to get you to a point that you are on a "maintenance" program rather than an endless "treatment" program, as is often the case with conventional methods. They will encourage your full participation in this endeavor, and tell you that results depend on your actions too. If they are knowledgeable and skilled, they have a clear understanding that it is your body that ultimately must heal itself, and that their therapy – while incredibly useful for providing conditions under which the body can heal – cannot cure you. Perhaps the biggest difference on the whole between natural and conventional therapies is that when performed by competent and qualified professionals, natural therapies will almost always help and rarely if ever hurt your condition.

Is There Another Solution to Arthritis?

Our current arthritis treatment paradigm is locked into a model that creates patients for life out of people suffering from arthritis symptoms. It relies exclusively on a variety of expensive, toxic medications to ease pain and temporarily retard tissue destruction, and even more expensive joint replacement surgery when patients believe there is nothing more that can be done. Arthritis is big business. NSAIDs are some of the top selling products for the pharmaceutical companies, and the industry relies heavily on arthritis sufferers for a steady income stream. Maintaining profits is a powerful incentive for the companies and professionals that prey on the unsuspecting, trusting patient by shamelessly or unknowingly keeping natural treatment therapies off the radar for those suffering with joint pain and dysfunction.

The popular nutraceuticals glucosamine and chondroitin have finally been accepted by mainstream healthcare providers and are commonly recommended as an adjunct to help maintain cartilage. Many doctors, in my view, perceive a threat and have consequently been highly critical of other successful natural preventions and remedies. Although largely ridiculed and dismissed by modern medicine altogether, there is a growing body of new evidence (even though empirical evidence has existed for centuries) that a radical diet change along with exercise can actually provide a superior alternative to unnecessary and harmful drugs. Because joint destruction appears to be caused primarily by inflammation and oxidative stress, antioxidants and foods (such as fruits and vegetables) that lower arachidonic acid can be the key to turning off – or more to the point – preventing the inflammatory cascade. This goes a long way in maintaining cartilage and bone health so that arthritis doesn't develop, or doesn't progress.

Our current arthritis treatment paradigm is locked into a model that creates patients for life out of people suffering from arthritis symptoms.

The common "wisdom" holds that diet has no effect on arthritis. Studies funded by industry continue to conclude that foods make no difference in alleviating the symptoms of any type of arthritis. The Arthritis Foundation, for example, goes so far as to say, "Because dietary management of gout is so restrictive and of limited benefit, medication is the best way to treat gout."[153] In actuality, quite the opposite has proven to be true in the few independent studies that have examined the subject: diet has been shown to be of utmost importance in causing, halting, and reversing the disease. Symptoms of osteoarthritis, rheumatoid arthritis and gout can be alleviated and often reversed by adopting a vegetarian or vegan diet that incorporates high levels of anti-inflammatory and antioxidant-rich foods.[154] In the case of gout, and as we covered before, it is critical to avoid high purine foods, especially meats, fish, caffeine, and alcohol, as well as sugar in order to halt the inflammatory process initiated by uric acid. In rheumatoid arthritis, it is likewise crucial to avoid animal proteins and processed foods, known for inciting the damaging immune process that causes the body to destroy its own healthy tissue.[155]

There has been significant anecdotal evidence over the years that avoiding meat, dairy, eggs and processed foods can bring enormous relief to rheumatoid arthritis sufferers and, in fact, halt the disease and restore functionality. As far back as 1973, Dr. Colin Dong, a California physician, successfully cured his own arthritis by adopting what he referred to as a Chinese peasant diet. He wrote two books about the benefits of eating rice, vegetables, nuts, seeds, and a little fish, while forbidding meat, dairy, soft drinks, alcohol, and all additives and chemicals.

Joint function is maximized with a diet high in antioxidants, high in omega-3 fatty acids, low in omega-6 fatty acids, and rich in nutrients supplied by greens, grains, legumes, fruit, and other whole plant foods.

Research from the early 1990s showed that certain oils, fish, and fresh vegetables were commonly associated with improvements while red meat, white flour, and soft drinks aggravated symptoms. A number of promising recent studies show that adopting a low-fat vegan diet can immediately reduce symptoms of pain, swelling and limited range of motion. One group of researchers from Norway did a controlled study in a supervised setting whereby a group of rheumatoid arthritis sufferers began the program with a 7- to 10-day fast. After the fast, half the group was assigned to a vegetarian diet, and the other half resumed their normal diet. They found significant improvement in the vegetarian group, and especially in the participants who chose to continue the diet beyond the clinical study. There are more studies indicating the benefits of a vegetarian lifestyle, including fasting, related to the prevention and eradication of arthritis. Joel Fuhrman, M.D. – a leading proponent of the vegetarian diet – monitored over 500 fasts in a variety of clinical conditions, followed by a vegan diet.

He reported in *Alternative Therapies* journal that fasting can offer both reduction in pain and lower inflammatory markers in patients with autoimmune illnesses, including rheumatoid arthritis. He also found that if the fasting period is extended long enough, a substantial number of patients actually experience total remission of autoimmune symptoms that do not return in about half of the cases.[156] John McDougall, M.D., a well-known author, physician and board certified internist whose philosophy is that degenerative disease can be prevented and treated with a plant-based diet of whole, unprocessed, low-fat foods, has had notable success in treating sufferers of rheumatoid arthritis with the McDougall diet, a vegan diet based in unprocessed plant foods and whole grains.[157-159] As mentioned earlier, the conclusion of T. Colin Campbell, Ph.D.'s *China Study* is that people who ate a diet low in animal proteins were the healthiest and lived the longest lives. Correspondingly, in 2002, there was a comparative study done between elderly in China – where the prevailing diet consists mostly of fruits and vegetables, rice and other grains, and fish – and the U.S. for hip osteoarthritis. The conclusion of the study was that the Chinese experienced hip osteoarthritis 80-90% less frequently than Caucasians in the United States.[160]

It should be apparent by now that to maintain joints it is necessary to avoid the Standard American Diet. Joint function is maximized with a diet high in antioxidants, high in omega-3 fatty acids, low in omega-6 fatty acids, and rich in nutrients supplied by greens, grains, legumes, fruit, and other whole plant foods. Likewise, it is crucial to avoid those foods that cause inflammation, such as meat, dairy, eggs, high fructose corn syrup, unhealthy fats, white flour and processed foods. The evidence is overwhelming that the weight gain associated with the Standard American Diet is a recipe for disaster: it is guaranteed to cause a condition of chronic inflammation in the body, which will certainly lead to ill health and a variety of the lifestyle diseases, including arthritis.

Your mental position about life and any health challenge is potentially the most essential aspect in determining your ability to recover health.

The Mindset of Health

While the quality of what we put into our bodies along with proper and consistent exercise are essential for good health, there is one thing that cannot be missing if we want true and lasting health – *a positive mindset, which includes an orientation toward health rather than disease.* Ralph Waldo Emerson said: "Nothing great was ever achieved without enthusiasm." Along these same lines, Abraham Lincoln said: "Determine that the thing can and shall be done, and then we shall find the way."

Your mental position about life and any health challenge is potentially the most essential aspect in determining your ability to recover health. My colleague Luann Pennesi, R.N., M.S., Director of Metropolitan Wellness, tells each one of her clients "Do not personalize disease, which means do not lose your identity to it. Disease can be temporary when we understand what our body is aiming to tell us, and then [we can] take positive actions to give it what it needs to heal itself." Positive, focused thinking, indeed, is what will enable you to embrace, as well as direct and sustain actions toward a new and healthy lifestyle, like the ones offered in this book. What we are presenting here is not just a way to deal with your arthritis and other diseases, it is a way of living that will enable you to eradicate these diseases while minimizing your risk of future illnesses for life. If this is of interest to you, then you will adopt an "I can" attitude; and it will guide you to make the choices that are essential for a joyful, fulfilling life free from chronic disease.

Science abounds in support of how our thoughts affect our biology. As we have established in the previous section on stress, if you are worried, stressed, and fearful much of the time, your body's functions, including your immune system, are being compromised. Not only this, but it may determine whether you manifest an illness related to a genetic predisposition. A study conducted by Massachusetts General Hospital and the Genomics Center at Beth Israel Deaconess Medical Centers found that the mind can actively turn on and turn off genes. "Now we've found how changing the activity of the mind can alter the way basic genetic instructions are implemented," stated Harvard Medical School professor Herbert Benson, M.D., co-senior author of the report. The study reported significant differences in the expressions of more than 2,200 genes between meditators and non-meditators. Some of these genes included those responsible for inflammation, the handling of free radicals, and programmed cell death, which can keep genetically impaired cells from turning into cancers.[161] This is an incredibly valuable finding for people suffering from any disease, including arthritis. Reporting on the same study, the Washington Post noted that researchers involved in the study said "they've taken a significant stride forward in understanding how relaxation techniques such as meditation, prayer and yoga improve health: by changing patterns of gene activity that affect how the body responds to stress." These mind-body practices as well as others have been used worldwide for millennia to prevent

A study conducted by Massachusetts General Hospital and the Genomics Center at Beth Israel Deaconess Medical Centers found that the mind can actively turn on and turn off genes.

and treat disease, and to promote wellness; this study provides the first compelling evidence that they affect gene expression changes in practitioners.[162]

Chronic physical pain very often leads to chronic anxiety and depression, which means that you want to do everything in your power to prevent or reverse this disorder. The emotional pain of arthritis is tremendous; it can cause you to withdraw, lose hope and not want to live, which is so far from how well we can live with the proper care. To make and sustain change, we must first become aware of the possibility of living a fulfilled life, which is one of the purposes of this book. Then, we must feel our desire enough to make the commitment to a different reality. The commitment is one

> Our unconscious mind has tremendous influence (more than we know) over our actions.

of heart and mind, it takes both. But the mind is incredibly powerful, and can oftentimes override our heart, so we must first understand it, and then learn how to deal with it in order to succeed in creating change. Simply put, we have the conscious mind and subconscious mind (typically termed the "unconscious" in scientific circles). The conscious mind is responsible for logic and reasoning while the subconscious mind, according to Sigmund Freud, is a repository for socially unacceptable ideas, wishes or desires, traumatic memories, and painful emotions. While the subconscious has largely been thought of as the receptacle for negative thoughts and experiences put out of mind by the mechanism of psychological repression, its contents do not necessarily have to be solely negative.[163] The key realization, however, is that in the common psychoanalytic view, the unconscious (comprised of both the personal unconsciousness and the collective unconsciousness, defined as the unconsciousness of humanity) is a *force* that can only be recognized by its effects, or the symptoms (or realities) it produces.

While this is a rudimentary definition for an extremely complex field of understanding, we need only to know this: Our unconscious mind has tremendous influence (more than we know) over our actions. When "sabotage patterns," for example, surface, we can use the power of our *conscious* mind to make the correct choices based on our commitment. How do we do this? By *imagining* what life would be like if we fall back into our same "old" patterns, and then actually *feeling* the painful feelings associated with these old ways. If we spend just enough time doing this, we will not want to engage in our old behaviors. Then, we can engage ourselves in imagining how much better life is and will be once we are relieved of the arthritis symptoms. Feel the positive feelings associated with the freedom of healthy living; these will keep you on track. If you slip up, simply refocus and reconnect to your commitment. Applying this level of awareness and consciousness to our efforts in creating a healthier existence makes it significantly easier to make better choices in the moment, which is actually all that is required. We create health for the future by making good choices now.

Much of your success will be determined by your ability to support yourself mentally and emotionally, which means structuring your time to support your new habits, eliminating toxic habits and relationships, doing more things that make you truly happy, letting go of beliefs that no longer serve you, and learning the art of self-love. As I said, this is a complex landscape to navigate, but one worthy of your attention and efforts. Consider seeking the help of coaches, spiritual teachers, and supportive friends and family to provide encouragement to you on this important journey. Also, visit Section III of this book for other recommended practices.

The Importance of Exercise

Patients are almost never advised to build up the muscles around a problem joint, but evidence shows that when a strength training program is instituted along with proper dietary changes, often symptoms resolve with no need for medication or surgery. The CDC says that "physical activity can reduce pain and improve function, mobility, mood, and quality of life for most adults with many types of arthritis including osteoarthritis, rheumatoid arthritis, fibromyalgia, and lupus." They also report that "scientific studies have shown that participation in moderate-intensity, low-impact physical activity several times a week improves pain, function, mood, and quality of life without worsening symptoms or disease severity."[164]

Unfortunately, most Americans have a sedentary lifestyle, and our leg, arm, back and stomach muscles frequently become weak from lack of use. Joint health is not possible without proper muscular support; diet alone cannot rehabilitate joints that have become impaired. All forms of exercise, including aerobic, muscle strengthening (resistance), and movement that promotes flexibility (such as yoga or stretching), are all relevant because they keep joints fully mobile while transporting nutrients and waste products to and from the cartilage to regulate and control joint swelling and pain. Strengthening the surrounding muscles also helps decrease bone loss and increases bone density, which supports the joints in proper functioning by protecting them from the pressure of carrying the weight of the body.

Not enough that can be said about the overriding value of exercise in creating and maintaining a healthy life. Energy and stamina are enhanced through exercise, which also decreases fatigue and improves the quality of sleep, which is an essential component of weight management. When we are tired and not sleeping well, we often gravitate toward foods that give us quick energy – typically sugary, calorie-dense processed foods with deleterious side effects. Regular exercise combats fatigue while regulating our appetite, inspiring us to make healthier food choices. For these reasons and more, exercise has been shown to enhance weight loss and promote long-term weight management, especially in those with arthritis who are overweight. As we've learned,

"**P**hysical activity can reduce pain and improve function, mobility, mood, and quality of life for most adults with many types of arthritis including osteoarthritis, rheumatoid arthritis, fibromyalgia, and lupus."

– *The Centers for Disease Control and Prevention*

lowering body weight decreases the forces on the joints, which is essential for those suffering with arthritis, and any other ailment for that matter. The bottom line is that obesity shortens life. Recent studies have linked every 10lbs of excess body weight to 1 year off your life expectancy.[165]

Exercise may offer additional benefits to improving or modifying arthritis. It has been proven to help lower the stress that causes us to tighten muscles, clench our jaws, and develop damaging muscle spasms. Strengthening muscles, while also developing flexibility through exercises such as swimming, power walking, dance, yoga or Pilates, helps to reduce tension, allowing the joints to move more freely. Of course, swimming is an excellent form of exercise for anyone suffering from arthritis and or obesity; it is easy on the joints and offers excellent cardio fitness while increasing muscle and bone strength. While exercising arthritic joints may seem counterintuitive, there is nothing that can help more than proper movement, along with a healthy diet. You will be astonished with the results when making these two changes alone. Ultimately, the only way to restore lost function is to provide circumstances that promote proper function, not to cover up the symptoms with drugs that are not designed to address the cause of the loss of function.

If there ever was a time to take action to become lighter; it is now! Ask yourself: Can I honestly afford to *wait* to make changes that could help me feel better today? Most importantly, make sure to choose exercise that is preferably near your home or workplace and that you enjoy; it is easier to stick with an exercise program that you like. Also, be sure to consult qualified physical trainers or professionals with expertise prior to beginning any kind of training program, especially weight training. One of the key aspects of joint health is correct alignment, and unless we receive instruction on proper form in the performance of any exercise we run the risk of damaging our joints rather than helping them. Please make sure to read the specific eating plan and exercise guidelines that we have outlined for you in Section II & III of this book. You will find them helpful in creating your personalized exercise and eating program.

A New Paradigm

In many ways, it is abundantly clear that for all intents and purposes the food corporations, the pharmaceutical companies, and our legislators have declared war on the American public. Whether they are unconscious of their actions, purposefully indifferent or simply ignorant of how to create health, they continue to fight tooth and nail to keep insular structures and systems in place – the very act of which brainwashes most of us into believing that we have few-to-no options for disease eradication other than what they are presenting. In particular, it is most disconcerting that the majority of elected and appointed government officials who we entrust, charter, and pay with our hard-earned tax dollars to protect us from corporate interests are doing just the opposite, and protecting – to our peril – their personal interests instead. Our expensive and costly modern medical system, built and run by mainly power-hungry individuals who by definition are more interested in protecting their positions (financial and otherwise) than in *"first, doing no harm,"* will *not* produce the type of care providers that can effect real change. Nor will government officials assigned to regulate the various factions within the industry be effective in dealing with them, or the medical problems of our time, when they are beholden to these groups for their own financial and political security and gain. Money – above all else – will keep this monstrous mechanism in place, and have us tethered to the medical establishment for life, unless more of us take charge of our health.

Adding to the challenge of change is the fact that the food industry simply doesn't want you to make healthy changes. Billions, if not trillions, of dollars are at stake – approximately 36 to 40 billion dollars would be lost by the food industry if each of us simply reduced our daily caloric intake by only 100 calories. This is about 4 potato chips, ¼ of a candy bar, and ¹/₃ of a soda. That's a large financial impact for a remarkably small shift in one lifestyle choice. It should be no wonder then why "food" companies forge ahead, keeping us fat, arthritic, in pain and addicted rather than leading the way toward healthier eating.[166] But we can no longer deny that our diet is ruining our health and that of our children, and the chance for a healthy future, for us, our country and our planet. We are already seeing the effects of toxic living in us and around us. What

Our expensive and costly modern medical system, built and run by mainly power-hungry individuals who by definition are more interested in protecting their positions (financial and otherwise) than in "first, doing no harm," will not produce the type of care providers that can effect real change.

does it take for us to pause and look? For the first time in recorded human history, *children* are suffering from lifestyle-based illnesses that are not necessarily related to poverty. Yes, our children are now suffering from arthritis, hypertension, heart disease and diabetes in record numbers. In truth, we all need to change, and we will have no future – unless something significant does change.

For the wise few in government and industry that follow a higher moral compass, and for those of you who will take the information in this book to heart and do whatever you can to create a healthier way of living, I honor you. Only those who are able to take an honest look at what is not working, who are able to ask and reflect upon the deeper questions, and then take appropriate actions will thrive. While it won't be easy at times, I can assure you that it will be worth it. The smiles that we see on people's faces when they make these changes and release their need, for example, for a cane, a cupcake or other physical or emotional support is truly inspiring.

My colleague Luanne Pennesi, R.N., M.S who assisted me with the arthritis study you will read about in the next section said: "What I witnessed after four weeks of people integrating this protocol into their lives was nothing short of miraculous. As a registered nurse, trained for 36 years to make sure that patients got their drugs, I could not believe what I was witnessing. Some were no longer using walkers or canes; I was truly amazed! This is what should be on the front pages of the *New York Times*, *USA Today, Time* magazine and every medical journal in America." When I see the results of this protocol in action – as I have recently – it's hard for me to believe that the majority of Americans have given up on their precious health for a few candies, cookies, sodas, meatball sandwiches, hot dogs and pizzas. Are we truly unwilling to take the necessary steps to change? And why don't we make better choices with respect to our physical well-being? The short answer is that we perceive change to be difficult and painful. Before you accept this as true, however, you may want to consider that a change may actually be less painful – and potentially even joyful – to what you are currently experiencing. Beginning on page115, we share results from our study of nearly 50 people actively affected by arthritis who participated in the protocol I am outlining in this book. You will read testimonies from people who have embraced my lifestyle recommendations and, as a result, are now living happier lives than they could have imagined, and with much less pain.

As I have shown you here, the reasons for arthritis are as numerous as its symptoms: our toxic foods, our lack of physical movement, our jobs, televisions, computers, smart phones and videogames all promote a sedentary lifestyle. We travel by car just to go a few blocks, we rely on "others" (doctors and pharmaceuticals) to make us well rather than finding out and taking steps to create a healthier life for ourselves, and we haven't learned how to manage the constant milieu of mental, emotional and physical stress. While we didn't get where we are completely on our own, it is entirely up to us whether we develop arthritis, or whether our current arthritis and pain worsens. We have *another choice* – to develop the determination to seek out enough information and support to make changes so that we become unflappable in the face of temptations, corporate agendas, Madison Avenue spin

W e have *another* choice – to develop the determination to seek out enough information and support to make changes so that we become unflappable in the face of temptations, corporate agendas, Madison Avenue spin masters, and the ill-informed physicians that are contributing to our nation's bleak health status.

masters, and the ill-informed physicians that are contributing to our nation's bleak health status. This choice is a commitment to doing something different, something truly empowering. We have seen what conventional medicine has to offer for joint damage, and the overwhelming evidence is that it will worsen our condition.

If you believe in your body's natural capacity to be strong and self-repairing, and you truly want to rid yourself from the pain associated with tissue degeneration, then you will find the motivation to do what you need to do. I've seen it a thousand times over: people changing their minds (first) and then their bodies for the better. As soon as enough of us do this, our family, friends and communities will follow; and so will others around the globe. As American cultural anthropologist Margret Mead said: "Never doubt for a moment that a small group of people can change the world, indeed they are the only ones that ever do."

Trust me when I tell you that the miracle of a healthy, pain-free body is not only possible, but probable if you follow these guidelines. As you continue to read on, you will learn about some of the people who are inspiring themselves (and others) to lead a better life. I encourage you to take the time to read what happened for these folks in just *three short weeks*. I can also share with you that there is hardly anything more worthwhile than bearing witness to the complete transformation of a human being who at one point in their life is constrained by their illness, and then shortly thereafter becomes free from arthritis and pain, and lives a life that they love. This is not only possible for you, but probable – if you follow the recommendations in this book. Then, you would have the distinction of being a member of a growing group of individuals who are triumphing over arthritis and pain *for life*. This really *is* something to celebrate!

Bibliography, Section I

1   The Heavy Burdern of Arthritis in the U.S. *The Arthritis Foundation* www.arthritis.org/media/newsroom/Arthritis_Prevalence_Fact_Sheet_5-31-11.pdf. Accessed 4/10/2012.

2   Arthritis - At A Glance. *Centers for Disease Control and Prevention* http://www.cdc.gov/chronicdisease/resources/publications/AAG/arthritis.htm accessed 10/5/12.

3   Lazar K. What a Pain. *The Boston Globe* Oct 19, 2009; http://www.boston.com/news/health/articles/2009/10/19/could_there_be_an_epidemic_of_osteoarthritis_in_our_future/, . Accessed 4/10/2012.

4   Hwang EJ, etal. Lived experience of Korean women suffering from rheumatoid arthritis: a phenomenological approach. *International Journal of Nursing Studies* 2004;41(3):239-246.

5   The Heavy Burdern of Arthritis in the U.S. *The Arthritis Foundation* www.arthritis.org/media/newsroom/Arthritis_Prevalence_Fact_Sheet_5-31-11.pdf. Accessed 4/10/2012.

6   The Heavy Burdern of Arthritis in the U.S. *The Arthritis Foundation* www.arthritis.org/media/newsroom/Arthritis_Prevalence_Fact_Sheet_5-31-11.pdf. Accessed 4/10/2012.

7   Osteoarthritis Fact Sheet 2008. *The Arthritis Foundation* www.arthritis.org/media/newsroom/.../Osteoarthritis_fact_sheet.pdf. Accessed 4/30/2012.

8   Arthritis- At A Glance. *Centers for Disease Control and Prevention* http://www.cdc.gov/chronicdisease/resources/publications/AAG/arthritis.htm accessed 10/5/12.

9   American Family Farmers Feed 155 People Each - 2% Americans Farm. suite101.com/article/american-family-farmers-feeds-155-people-each-2-americans-farm-a231011 Accessed 10/5/12.

10 Haupt A. Health Buzz: Many U.S. Workers Sleep-Deprived. health.usnews.com/health-news/articles/2012/04/27/health-buzz-many-us-workers-sleep-deprived Accessed 10/5/2012.

11 Black A. Unnecessary surgery exposed! Why 60% of all surgeries are medically unjustified and how surgeons exploit patients to generate profits. October 07, 2005 http://www.naturalnews.com/012291_unnecessary_surgery_hysterectomies.html. Accessed 10/5/2012.

12   Kliff S. Why would hospitals like HCA perform unnecessary surgery? Because it pays. *Washington Post* 8/7/2012; http://www.washingtonpost.com/blogs/ezra-klein/wp/2012/08/07/why-would-hospitals-like-hca-perform-unnecessary-surgery-because-it-pays/. Accessed 10/5/2012.

13   Musemeche C. Childhood obesity leads to unnecessary surgeries. *The New York Times blogs* 4/25/2012; http://parenting.blogs.nytimes.com/2012/04/25/childhood-obesity-leads-to-unnecessary-surgeries/. Accessed 10/5/2012.

14   Elliott VS. More Than Half of Surgeries are Outpatient. 3/24/2010; http://www.ama-assn.org/amednews/2010/03/22/bisc0324.htm. Accessed 5/4/2010.

15   LRP-Publications. Physician-owned surgery centers come under researchers' scrutiny. *Risk & Insurance* 6/10/2012, http://www.riskandinsurance.com/story.jsp?storyId=533348862. Accessed 10/5/2012.

16   Cullen KA, Hall MJ, Golosinskiy A. *Ambulatory Surgery in the United States, 2006.* National Health Statistics Reports, no. 11;2009.

17   PR-Newswire. Total knee and hip replacement surgery projections show meteoric rise by 2030. *PR-Newswire* 3/24/2012; http://www.prnewswire.com/news-releases/total-knee-and-hip-replacement-surgery-projections-show-meteoric-rise-by-2030-55519727.html. Accessed 10/5/2012.

18   Marchione M. Joint Replacements for Baby Boomers. *The Huffington Post* 5/23/2011; http://www.huffingtonpost.com/2011/05/23/joint-replacement-knee-hip-surgery-baby-boomers_n_865368.html. Accessed 10/6/2012.

19   Null G., Feldman M., Rasio D., Dean C. *Death by Medicine.* Mount Jackson, VA: Praktikos Books; 2011.

20   O'Reilly KB. Chronic pain costs U.S. $635 billion a year. amednews.com 2011; www.ama-assn.org/*amednews*/2011/07/04/prsr0708.htm Accessed 10/5/12.

21   Longley R. Almost Half of Americans Take at Least One Prescription Drug: Half of elderly take more. *about.com* http://usgovinfo.about.com/od/healthcare/a/usmedicated.htm. Accessed 10/5/2012.

22   United States Health. *Centers for Disease Control and Prevention* 2011; www.cdc.gov/nchs/data/hus/hus11.pdf#glance. Accessed 10/5/2012.

23   Lazarou, etal. Incidence of Adverse Drug Reactions in Hospitalized Patients. *JAMA.* 279(15):1200-1205.

24   Young T. Facts on Prescription Drug Deaths and the Drug Industry *The Conference* http://theconference.ca/facts-on-prescription-drug-deaths-and-the-drug-industry. Accessed 10/5/2012.

25   Avila J, Murray M. Prescription painkiller use at record high for Americans. *abcnews.com* 4/20/2011; http://abcnews.go.com/US/prescription-painkillers-record-number-americans-pain-medication/story?id=13421828#.UJWwl4YUocc. Accessed 10/5/2012.

26   Trade secrets: Chemical body burden. *PBS: Public Broadcasting Service* http://www.pbs.org/tradesecrets/problem/bodyburden.html# Accessed 10/5/2012.

27   BodyBurden2-Thepollutioninnewborns.*EnvironmentalWorkingGroup* http://www.ewg.org/reports/bodyburden2/execsumm.php. Accessed 10/5/2012.

28   Federal Employees Health Benefits Program: Frequently Asked Questions. *U.S. Office of Personnel Management* http://www.opm.gov/insure/archive/health/qa/qa.asp?rx Accessed 10/5/2012.

29   Connor S, Glaxo Chief: Our Drugs do not Work on Most Patients, *The Independent,* September 8, 2003, http://www.independent.co.uk/news/science/glaxo-chief-our-drugs-do-not-work-on-most-patients-575942.html Accessed 11/29/12.

30   The benefits of personalized medicine. *The Jackson Laboratory* http://genetichealth.jax.org/personalized-medicine/what-is/benefits.html Accessed 10/5/2012.

31   Why are drug costs on the rise? *U.S. Office of Personnel Management* http://www.opm.gov/insure/health/faq/rx.asp. Accessed 10/5/12.

32   Food and Drug Administration. *Wikipedia.* Accessed 10/5/12.

33   Angell M. *The truth about the drug companies: How they deceive us and what to do about it.* New York: Random House; 2004.

34   Blackburn H. *Overview: The Seven Countries Study in Brief.* School of Public Health: University of Minnesota.

35   Campbell TC, Campbell TM. *The China Study: The most comprehensive study of nutrition ever conducted and the startling implications for diet, weight loss and long-term health.* Dallas, TX: BenBella Books; 2005.

36   Belluck P. Children's Life Expectancy Being Cut Short by Obesity. *The New York Times.* Mar 17, 2005. Accessed 4/28/2012.

37   Osteoarthritis. *About.com* 2004; http://adam.about.net/reports/000035_4.htm. Accessed 5/12/2012.

38   Doheny K. Arthritis Patients More Likely to be Obese. *WebMD Arthritis and Joint Pain Center* http://arthritis.webmd.com/news/20110428/arthritis-patients-more-likely-be-obese. Accessed 10/5/2012.

39   How Does Inequality Define the Health of a Nation? *yesmagazine.org* http://www.yesmagazine.org/happiness/how-does-inequality-define-the-health-of-a-nation?utm_source=wkly20120727&utm_medium=email&utm_campaign=mrVideo. Accessed 10/5/2012.

40   Arthritis. *Pub Med Health* Feb 14, 2011; http://www.ncbi.nlm.nih.gov/pubmedhealth/PMH0002223/. Accessed 5/3/2012.

41   Schneider M, etal. *The Handbook of Self-Healing.* Penguin; 1994.

42   Osteoarthritis *about.com* 2004; http://adam.about.net/reports/000035_4.htm. Accessed 5/12/2012.

43   Sturmer T, etal. Severity and Extent of Osteoarthritis and Low Grade Systemic Inflammation as Assessed by High Sensitivity C Reactive Protein. *Annals of the Rheumatic Diseases.* 2004;63(2):200-205.

44   Hauser R. The Acceleration of Articular Cartilage Degeneration in Osteoarthritis by Nonsteroidal Anti-inflammatory Drugs, Journal of Prolotherapy. *Journal of Prolotherapy.* 2010;2(1):305-322.

45   Lu YC. *In Vitro Models of Cartilage Degradation Following Joint Injury: Mechanical Overload, Inflammatory Cytokines and Therapeutic Approaches.* Boston: Biological Engineering, Massachusetts Institute of Technology; 2010.

46   McCarty M. Nutraceutical Strategies for Preserving Cartilage in Osteoarthritis, NutriGuard Research. http://catalyticlongevity.org/prepub_archive/nutraceuticals-OA[1][1][1][1][1][1][1][1].pdf. Accessed 10/5/2012.

47   Sturmer T, etal. Severity and Extent of Osteoarthritis and Low Grade Systemic Inflammation as Assessed by High Sensitivity C Reactive Protein. *Annals of the Rheumatic Diseases.* 2004;63(2):200-205.

48   Andrews T. A List of NSAIDs. *Livestrong.com, The Lance Armstrong Foundation* Mar 28, 2011; http://www.livestrong.com/article/99121-list-nsaids/. Accessed 4/28/2012.

49   Eustice C. Gastrointestinal Bleeding - Don't Ignore Your Symptoms. *about. com* Jul 14, 2008; http://arthritis.about.com/od/azdrugsideeffects1/a/ GI_bleeding.htm. Accessed 5/2/2012.

50   Wolfe M, etal. Gastrointestinal Toxicity of Nonsteroidal Antiinflammatory Drugs. *New England Journal of Medicine.* Jun 17, 1999;340(24).   http://aramis.stanford.edu/downloads/GI..NSAID. pdf. Accessed 5/3/2012.

51   Presley H. Vioxx and the Merck Team Effort. *The Kenan Institute for Ethics at Duke University* 2009; http://www.duke.edu/web/ kenanethics/CaseStudies/Vioxx.pdf. Accessed 3/5/2012.

52   Lanza F. A Guideline for the Treatment and Prevention of NSAID-Induced Ulcers. *The American Journal of Gastroenterology.* 1998; 93(11).

53   Silverman E. Merck Wins Reversal in A Vioxx Lawsuit. *Pharmalot* Aug 29, 2011; http://www.pharmalot.com/2011/08/merck-wins-32m-reversal-in-vioxx-case/. Accessed 4/28/2012.

54   *Celebrex Heart Dangers:* CBS Evening News; Dec 22, 2004.

55   *Analysis and recommendations for Agency action regarding non-steroidal anti-inflammatory drugs and cardiovascular risk.* Food and Drug Administration;Apr 6, 2005.

56   Selvan T, etal. A Clinical Study on Glucosamine Sulfate versus Combination of Glucosamine Sulfate and NSAIDs in Mild to Moderate Knee Osteoarthritis. *Scientific World Journal.* Apr 1, 2012. Accessed 5/12/2012.

57   Vijayan S, etal. Autologous chondrocyte implantation for osteochondral lesions in the knee using a bilayer collagen membrane and bone graft: a two- to eight-year follow-up study. *The Journal of Bone and Joint Surgery, British Volume.* Apr 2012;94(4):488-492. http:// www.ncbi.nlm.nih.gov/pubmed/22434464. Accessed 5/1/2012.

58   Zaslav K, Cole B, Brewster R, et al. A Prospective Study of Autologous Chondrocyte Implantation in Patients With Failed Prior Treatment for Articular Cartilage Defect of the Knee: Results of the Study of the Treatment of Articular Repair (STAR) Clinical Trial *The American Journal of Sports Medicine.* 2008;37(1):42-55.

59   Types of Replacement Parts. *The Arthritis Foundation* 2012; http:// www.arthritis.org/types-replacement-parts.php. Accessed 5/15/2012.

60   Ng N. Range Of Motion Of The Knee. *livestrong.com* http://www.livestrong.com/article/345122-range-of-motion-of-the-knee/. Accessed 10/5/2012.

61   Concerns about Metal-on-Metal Hip Implant Systems. *Food and Drug Administration* Mar 28, 2012; http://www.fda.gov/MedicalDevices /ProductsandMedicalProcedures/ImplantsandProsthetics /MetalonMetalHipImplants/ucm241604.htm. Accessed 5/10/2012.

62   NHS Choices, Fears of faulty 'toxic' hip replacement implant. *The National Health Service* Jan 30, 2010; http://www.nhs.uk/news/ 2012/01January/Pages/hip-implant-fears.aspx. Accessed 5/10/2012.

63   Cohen D. Hip Implants: How Safe is Metal on Metal?. *British Medical Journal.* Mar 2012;344(3). http://www.bmj.com/content/344/bmj. e1410. Accessed 5/10/2012.

64   Questions and Answers about Hip Replacement. *National Institute of Arthritis and Musculoskeletal and Skin Diseases* http://www.niams. nih.gov/Health_Info/Hip_Replacement/default.asp#8.   Accessed 10/5/2012.

65   Osteoarthritis - Surgery. *University of Maryland Medical Center* http:// www.umm.edu/patiented/articles/what_surgical_treatments_ osteoarthritis_000035_11.htm. Accessed 10/5/2012.

66   What are the risks and complications of hip replacement surgery? *American Association of Hip and Knee Surgeons* http://www.aahks. org/patients/documentary/inside_look.asp. Accessed 5/10/2012.

67   Osteoarthritis - Surgery. *University of Maryland Medical Center* http:// www.umm.edu/patiented/articles/what_surgical_treatments_ osteoarthritis_000035_11.htm. Accessed 10/5/2012.

68   Who Gets Rheumatoid Arthritis? *The Arthritis Foundation* 2012; http://www.arthritis.org/who-gets-rheumatoid-arthritis.php. Accessed 5/1/2012.

69   Woolf AD, Pfleger B. Burden of major musculoskeletal conditions. *World Health Organization* www.who.int/bulletin/volumes/81/9/ Woolf.pdf. Accessed 10/5/2012.

70   What is Rheumatoid Arthritis? *Web MD* http://www.webmd.com/ rheumatoid-arthritis/rheumatoid-arthritis-and-osteoporosis. Accessed 10/5/2012.

71 Weinblatt M. Rheumatoid Arthritis: More Aggressive Approach Improves Outlook. *Cleveland Clinic Medical Journal.* May 2004;71(5). http://www.ccjm.org/content/71/5/409.full.pdf. Accessed 4/30/2012.

72 Rheumatoid Arthritis. *Mayo Clinic* Nov 2, 2011; http://www.mayoclinic.com/health/rheumatoidarthritis/DS00020/DSECTION=symptoms. Accessed 5/2/2012.

73 What is Rheumatoid Arthritis? *National Institutes of Health Osteoporosis and Related Bone Diseases* Jan 2011; http://www.niams.nih.gov/health_info/bone/Osteoporosis/Conditions_Behaviors/osteoporosis_ra.asp, , 5/1/2012.

74 Abedin S. 10 Serious Rheumatoid Arthritis Symptoms. *WebMD* http://www.webmd.com/rheumatoid-arthritis/features/10-serious-rheumatoid-arthritis-symptoms. Accessed 10/5/2012.

75 Gonzalez A, etal. Mortality Trends in Rheumatoid Arthritis: The role of Rheumatoid Factor. *Journal of Rheumatology.* 2008;35(6):1009-1014. http://www.ncbi.nlm.nih.gov/pmc/articles/PMC2834198/pdf/nihms75088.pdf. Accessed 5/13/2012.

76 Osteoporosis. *Wikipedia.* Accessed 10/5/2012.

77 What is Rheumatoid Arthritis? *National Institutes of Health Osteoporosis and Related Bone Diseases* Jan 2011; http://www.niams.nih.gov/health_info/bone/Osteoporosis/Conditions_Behaviors/osteoporosis_ra.asp, , 5/1/2012.

78 Rheumatoid Arthritis. *University of Maryland Medical Center* 2011; http://www.umm.edu/altmed/articles/rheumatoid-arthritis-000142.htm. Accessed 5/15/2012.

79 The Biologics: Comparing Effectiveness, Safety, Side Effects, and Price, . *Consumer Reports Health* Jun 2010; http://www.consumerreports.org/health/resources/pdf/best-buy-drugs/BBD_Rheumatoid_Arthritis.pdf. Accessed 5/16/2012.

80 Rodan G. Mechanism of Action of Bisphosphonates. *Annual Review of Pharmacology and Toxicology,.* 38:375-388. http://www.annualreviews.org/doi/abs/10.1146/annurev.pharmtox.38.1.375. Accessed 4/28/2012.

81 Salari P, Abdollahi M. Long Term Bisphosphonate Use in Osteoporotic Patients; A Step Forward, Two Steps Back. *Journal of Pharmacy & Pharmaceutical Sciences.* 2012;15(2). http://ejournals.library.ualberta.ca/index.php/JPPS/article/view/12519. Accessed 4/30/2012.

82   Doherty M. New Insights into the Epidemiology of Gout. *Rheumatology.* 2009;48:ii2-ii8.

83   Murry R, etal. *Harper's Illustrated Biochemistry.* New York: McGraw-Hill Medical Publishing; 2012.

84   Zhu, etal. Prevalence of Gout and Hyperuricemia in the US General Population. *Arthritis & Rheumatism.* 2011.

85   Patterson E, etal. Health Implications of High Dietary Omega-6 Polyunsaturated Fatty Acids. *Journal of Nutrition and Metabolism.* 2012. http://www.hindawi.com/journals/jnume/2012/539426/. Accessed 5/5/2012.

86   Sturmer T, etal. Severity and Extent of Osteoarthritis and Low Grade Systemic Inflammation as Assessed by High Sensitivity C Reactive Protein. *Annals of Rheumatic Disease.* 2004;63(2):200-205.

87   Farah H, Buzby J. US Food Consumption up 16% since 1970. *Amber Waves, USDA* Nov 2005; http://www.ers.usda.gov/AmberWaves/November05/findings/usfoodconsumption.htm. Accessed 5/5/2012.

88   Patterson E, etal. Health Implications of High Dietary Omega-6 Polyunsaturated Fatty Acids. *Journal of Nutrition and Metabolism.* 2012. http://www.hindawi.com/journals/jnume/2012/539426/. Accessed 5/5/2012.

89   ibid.

90   *Lighten Up – Weighing in on the Weight Debate* [DVD]: VegSource; Oct 23, 2009.

91   Essential Fats in Food Oils. *National Institutes of Health* 2004; http://efaeducation.nih.gov/sig/esstable.html. Accessed 4/23/2012.

92   *From Oil to Nuts: The Essential Facts of Fats, Nuts, and Oil* [DVD]: VegSource; Jul 6, 2011.

93   Bartsch H, Nair J. Chronic inflammation and oxidative stress in the genesis and perpetuation of cancer: role of lipid peroxidation, DNA damage, and repair. *Langenbecks Archives for Surgery.* Sep 2006;391(5): 499-510. http://www.ncbi.nlm.nih.gov/pubmed/16909291. Accessed 5/15/2012.

94   Kim M, etal. Long-term vegetarians have low oxidative stress, body fat, and cholesterol levels. *Nutritional Research Practice.* 2012; 6 (2):155-161. http://www.ncbi.nlm.nih.gov/pmc/articles/PMC3349038/?tool=pubmed. Accessed 5/10/2012.

[95]   Hailu A, etal. Associations Between Meat Consumption and the Prevalence of Degenerative Arthritis and Soft Tissue Disorders in the Adventist Health Study, California, USA. *The Journal of Nutrition, Health & Aging.* Jan 2006. http://www.highbeam.com/doc/1P3-996177371. html. Accessed 5/12/2012.

[96]   Sabaté J, Wein M. Vegetarian Diets and Childhood Obesity. *American Journal of Clinical Nutrition.* 2010;91(5):15258-15298.

[97]   Meat eaters more likely to be obese than vegetarians. *News - Medical* Jun 27, 2005; http://www.news-medical.net/news/2005/06/27/11299. aspx. Accessed 5/10/2012.

[98]   Lang S. Eating Less Red Meat May Help Reduce Osteoporosis Risk, Studies Show. *Cornell Chronicles* 1996; http://www.news.cornell.edu/chronicle/96/11.14.96/osteoporosis.html. Accessed 5/15/2012.

[99]   Sellmeyer D, etal. A high ratio of dietary animal to vegetable protein increases the rate of bone loss and the risk of fracture in postmenopausal women. *American Journal of Clinical Nutrition.* 2001;73:118-122. Accessed 4/28/2012.

[100] Barzel U, Massey L. Excess Dietary Protein can Adversely Affect Bone. *Journal of Nutrition.* 1998;128(6):1051-1053.

[101] Fuhrman J. Super Immunity. *Harper One.* New York 2011.

[102] Barzel U, Massey L. Excess Dietary Protein can Adversely Affect Bone. *The Journal of Nutrition.* 1998;128(6):1051-1053.

[103] Prevalence of Obesity Among Adults with Arthritis -- United States, 2003-2009. *MMWR.* Apr 29, 2011;60(16):509-513. http://www.cdc.gov/mmwr/preview/mmwrhtml/mm6016a4.htm. Accessed 5/2/2012.

[104] Adult Obesity Facts. *Centers for Disease Control and Prevention* 2012; http://www.cdc.gov/obesity/data/adult.html. Accessed 10/10/2012.

[105] Aaboe J, etal. Effects of an intensive weight loss program on knee joint loading in obese adults with knee osteoarthritis. *Osteoarthritis and Cartilage.* 2011;19(7):822-828.

[106] Murphy L, etal. Lifetime risk of symptomatic knee osteoarthritis. *Arthritis and Rheumatism.* 2008;59(9):1207-1213.

[107] Stobbe M. Group Predicts Rapid Rise in Obesity in US. *washingtontimes. com* Sep 18, 2012; http://www.washingtontimes.com/news/2012/sep/18/group-predicts-rapid-rise-in-obesity-in-us/. Accessed 10/5/2012.

108 Schwarz SM. Obesity in Children. *Medscape Reference* http://emedicine. medscape.com/article/985333-overview. Accessed 10/5/2012.

109 Trasande L, Attina T, Blustein J. Association between urinary bisphenol A concentration and obesity prevalence in children and adolescents. *Journal of the American Medical Association.* 2012 Sep 19;308(11): 1113-1121.

110 *Weight of the Nation, Part I:* HBO Documentary Films; 2012.

111 The Fast Food Ban. *Eating Well* http://www.eatingwell.com/food_ news_origins/food_news/the_fast_food_ban. Accessed 11/1/2012.

112 Jackson A. *TheDiggerer.com* Mar 20, 2012; http://thediggerer.com/ index.php/component/k2/item/1-wv-legislature-bans-fast-food-drive-thru-windows. Accessed 10/5/2012.

113 Blodget H. Disney to Ban Junk-Food Ads for Kids as American Struggles with its Fat Problem. *Yahoo! Finance* Jun 5, 2012; http://finance.yahoo. com/blogs/daily-ticker/disney-ban-junk-food-ads-kids-america-struggles-165346887.html. Accessed 10/5/2012.

114 *Weight of the Nation, Part III:* HBO Documentary Films; 2012.

115 ibid.

116 Wartman K. Pizza is a Vegetable? Congress Defies Logic, Betrays our Children. *Huffington Post* Nov 18, 2011; http://www.huffingtonpost. com/kristin-wartman/pizza-is-a-vegetable_b_1101433.html. Accessed 10/5/2012.

117 ibid.

118 O'Connor A. Bans on School Junk Food Pay Off in California. *The New York Times blogs* May 8, 2012; http://well.blogs.nytimes.com/2012/05/08/ bans-on-school-junk-food-pay-off-in-california/. Accessed 10/5/2012.

119 McCullick B. UGA study: Physical education in schools not enough to combat obesity in most states. *The Red & Black* Jul 6, 2012; http:// www.redandblack.com/news/uga-physical-education-in-schools-not-enough-to-combat-obesity/article_9f58e648-c76a-11e1-af0f-001a4bcf6878.html. Accessed 10/5/2012.

120 *Journal of Teaching in Physical Education.*

121 Decline of Physical Activity. *pta.org* http://www.pta.org/topic_decline_ of_physical_activity.asp Accessed 10/5/2012.

[122] Entin E. Rethinking (Instead of Eliminating) Recess at Low-Income Schools. *The Atlantic* May 3, 2012; http://www.theatlantic.com/ health/archive/2012/05/rethinking-instead-of-eliminating-recess-at-low-income-schools/256679/. Accessed 10/5/2012.

[123] *The Association Between School-Based Physical Activity, Including Physical Education, and Academic Performance.* Atlanta, GA: U.S. Department of Health and Human Services, Centers for Disease Control and Prevention;2010.

[124] FTC Report Sheds New Light on Food Marketing to Children and Adolescents. *Federal Trade Commission* Jul 29, 2008; http://www. ftc.gov/opa/2008/07/foodmkting.shtm. Accessed 5/15/2012.

[125] Guterl F. Would You Like Fries with your Clone? *The Daily Beast (from Newsweek)* Jan 17, 2008; http://www.thedailybeast.com/newsweek/ 2008/01/17/would-you-like-fries-with-your-clone.html.

[126] Shut Up and Eat: The Beef Industry's Lawsuit Against Oprah Winfrey, Center for Media and Democracy. *PR Watch.* 1997;4(2). http://www. prwatch.org/prwissues/1997Q2/eat.html. Accessed 5/1/2012.

[127] Lesser L, etal. Relationship between Funding Source and Conclusion among Nutrition-Related Scientific Articles. *Plos Medicine.* 2007;4(1). http://www.plosmedicine.org/article/info:doi/10.1371/journal. pmed.0040005. Accessed 5/3/2012.

[128] Interagency Working Group on Food Marketed to Children, Preliminary Proposed Nutrition Principles to Guide Industry Self-Regulatory Efforts. Apr 28, 2011; https://docs.google.com /viewer?a=v&q=cache:FXVa7hq43OQJ:www.ftc.gov/os/2011/04/ 110428foodmarketproposedguide.pdf+interagency+working+ group+on+food+marketed+to+children&hl=en&gl=us&pid=bl& srcid=ADGEESi9BFNJUz2UWRxkk1lQxcZbuOTM9fvPBr8-_Mw_Nvv X5rLof3oUxIoO0LT-WgQp9CZ86_Fv5PZth9oa8R-ZkjP_Nw12695 n D J 6 G u 5 7 S J W A z 4 u c v 2 s e W M 9 2 g I a 5 r O 8 9 W 0 - h _ wSfZ&sig=AHIEtbS-owpXNDnRbG-i0TWFImSQIimn2g.   Accessed 5/14/2012.

[129] Watzman N. Congressional Letter Writing Campaign Helps Torpedo Voluntary Food Marketing Guidelines for Kids. *Sunlight Foundation* May 1, 2012; http://reporting.sunlightfoundation.com/2012/ congressional_letter_writing_campaign/. Accessed 5/5/2012.

130 Nestle M. Congress Caves in Again, Delays IWG Recommendations. *Food Politics.* Dec 17, 2011. http://www.foodpolitics.com/2011/12/congress-caves-in-again-delays-iwg-recommendations/.

131 Fuhrman J. Super Immunity. *Harper One.* New York 2011.

132 Sweetened Drinks Raise Women's Risk for Obesity, Type 2 Diabetes. *Harvard Medical School Family Health Guide* Dec 2004; http://www.health.harvard.edu/fhg/updates/update1204b.shtml. Accessed 5/6/2012.

133 Gearhardt A, etal. Preliminary validation of the Yale Food Addiction Scale. *Appetite.* 5/1/2012 2009;52(2):430-436.

134 Wang, Volkow N. Brain Dopamine and Obesity. *The Lancet.* Feb 3, 2001 2001;357.

135 Langreth R, Stanford D. Fatty Foods Addictive as Cocaine in Growing Body of Science. *Bloomberg News.* Nov 2, 2011. http://www.bloomberg.com/news/2011-11-02/fatty-foods-addictive-as-cocaine-in-growing-body-of-science.html.

136 Wang G, Volkow N, etal. Brain Dopamine and Obesity. *The Lancet.* Feb 3, 2001;357. http://www.ncbi.nlm.nih.gov/pubmed/11210998. Accessed 5/4/2012.

137 Fuhrman J. Super Immunity. *Harper One* New York 2011.

138 Liebman B. Food & Addiction, Can Some Foods Hijack the Brain?. *Nutrition Action Health Letter* May 2012.

139 Thompson PD, Buchner D, Piña IL, et al. Exercise and Physical Activity in the Prevention and Treatment of Atherosclerotic Cardiovascular Disease. *Circulation.* 2003;107:3109-3116.

140 Lovett K. Exercise and Disease Prevention. http://www.vanderbilt.edu/AnS/psychology/health_psychology/exercise.htm 10/5/2012.

141 *Weight of the Nation, Part II:* HBO Documentary Films; 2012.

142 ibid.

143 Stress Facts. *The Health Resource Network* http://www.stresscure.com/hrn/facts.html Accessed 10/5/2012.

144 ibid.

[145]   The Numbers Count: Mental Disorders in America. *National Institute of Mental Health* http://www.nimh.nih.gov/health/publications/the-numbers-count-mental-disorders-in-america/index.shtml. Accessed 10/5/2012.

[146]   ibid.

[147]   Bedson J, Croft P. The discordance between clinical and radiographic knee osteoarthritis: A systematic search and summary of the literature. *Musculoskeletal Disorders.* 2008;9(116).

[148]   Null, G, Reverse *Arthritis and Pain Naturally,* [DVD]. New York, NY, Gary Null & Associates, 2012.

[149]   Brownlee S. The Doctor Will See You - If You're Quick. *The Daily Beast (from Newsweek)* Apr 16, 2012; http://www.thedailybeast.com/newsweek/2012/04/15/why-your-doctor-has-no-time-to-see-you.html. Accessed 10/5/2012.

[150]   Torrey T. Why Is My Doctor in Such a Hurry? Why Won't He Spend Enough Time with Me? *about.com* Nov 14, 2008; http://patients.about.com/od/followthemoney/f/FAQdoctortime.htm.   Accessed 10/5/2012.

[151]   Reichenberg-Ullman J. Why Naturopathic Medicine is a Bargain. *healthy.net*http://www.healthy.net/Health/Article/Why_Naturopathic_Medicine_is_a_Bargain/624. Accessed 10/5/2012.

[152]   ibid.

[153]   Safe Foods for Gout. *The Arthritis Foundation* http://www.arthritis.org/foods-for-gout.php. Accessed 5/4/2012.

[154]   McCarty M. A Low-Fat, Whole-Food Vegan Diet, as well as Other Strategies That Down-Regulate IGF-1 Activity, May Slow the Human Aging Process. *Medical Hypothesis.* 2003;60(6):784-792. http://www.ncbi.nlm.nih.gov/pubmed/12699704. Accessed 5/4/2012.

[155]   Kjeldsen-Kragh J. Mediterranean Diet Intervention in Rheumatoid Arthritis. *Annals of Rheumatic Disease.* 2003;62:193-195. http://www.ncbi.nlm.nih.gov/pmc/articles/PMC1754473/. Accessed 5/5/2012.

[156]   Spotlight on Reversing and Preventing Arthritis. *DrFuhrman.com* http://www.drfuhrman.com/disease/arthritis.aspx. Accessed 10/5/2012.

[157] Lewenstein H. Diet & Arthritis – What You Eat and Don't Eat May Help Ease the Aches and Pain. *The Seattle Times.* Feb 21, 1996. http://community.seattletimes.nwsource.com/archive/?date= 19960221&slug=2315124, . Accessed 5/1/2012.

[158] Kjeldsen-Kragh J. Mediterranean Diet Intervention in Rheumatoid Arthritis *Annals of Rheumatic Disease.* 2003; 62:193-195. http:// www.ncbi.nlm.nih.gov/pmc/articles/PMC1754473/.   Accessed 5/5/2012.

[159] McDougall J, etal. Effects of a Very Low-Fat, Vegan Diet in Subjects with Rheumatoid Arthritis. *The Journal of Alternative and Complementary Medicine.* 2002;8(1):71-75. http://www.vegsource.com/articles/ McDougall_Arthritis.pdf. Accessed 4/30/2012.

[160] Nevitt MC, Xu L, Zhang Y, et al. Very low prevalence of hip osteoarthritis among Chinese elderly In Beijing, China, compared with whites in the United States: the Beijing osteoarthritis study. *pubmed.com.* 2002;46(7):1773-1779.   http://www.ncbi.nlm.nih.gov/pubmed/ 12124860. Accessed 10/5/2012.

[161] Blake T. Some Surprising Benefits of Meditation. *Kajama* http://www. kajama.com/index.php?file=articledetail&id=936FD18C-EB29- 4BA7-B83E-1FE277B39305&PageNum=1 Accessed 11/20/2012.

[162] Littman J. Finally -- Scientific Proof that Our Thoughts Affect Our Health. (We Already Knew That!). *Empower Network* Oct 15, 2012.

[163] Subconscious. *Wikipedia.* Accessed 10/5/2012.

[164] Physical Activity and Arthritis. The Centers for Disease Control and Prevention http://www.cdc.gov/arthritis/pa_overview.htm. Accessed 10/5/2012.

[165] Schneider M, etal. *The Handbook of Self-Healing.* Penguin; 1994.

[166] *Weight of the Nation, Part III:* HBO Documentary Films; 2012.

Section II

Clinical Study on the Effects of Nutrition

At Gary Null and Associates we were recently able to put our theories and research into practice with a clinical study in which we recruited subjects with varying degrees of osteoarthritis symptoms to study the effects of nutritional intervention and lifestyle changes. The following section demonstrates our results...

Nutrition Intervention Reverses Arthritis Symptoms

By Gary Null Ph.D., Martin Feldman M.D.,
and Luanne Pennesi R.N., M.S.

Abstract

Arthritis prevalence in the U.S. is substantial and predicted to increase. This study documents an intervention of lifestyle changes including diet, dietary supplements and exercise to address issues of pain relief and function for both rheumatoid and osteoarthritis. A vegan, gluten-free diet with daily exercise was taught with instruction in environmental hygiene, stress reduction and examination of beliefs and attitudes over a period of three weeks. A total of 43 subjects and 57 control subjects were used. Based on daily diaries and physical examinations the reports show a statistically significant improvement in all of the indices measured.

Introduction

For the years 2007-2009, U.S. prevalence of doctor diagnosed arthritis was 49.9 million persons or 22.2% of the adult population.[1] This is a sizeable increase from 37.9 million people, or 15% of the total U.S. population, in 1990.[2] By the year 2030, this figure is expected to increase to 67 million, or 25% of the adult population. At that time, 9.3% of the adult population or 25 million Americans are predicted to have arthritis-related activity limitations. Working age adults ages 45-64 years will account for one-third of arthritis cases.[3] Arthritis medications have dangerous side effects, including an estimated 16,500 annual U.S. deaths from non-steroidal anti-inflammatory medications for arthritis alone.[4] With these known dangers and the wide prevalence and associated pain and other consequences of arthritic conditions, finding an effective and safe alternative treatment would greatly benefit many.

Much of the protocol used for this study has had extensive scientific research showing positive outcomes for arthritic and other conditions related to inflammation such as diabetes, cancer, heart disease and Alzheimer's disease. This section will review historical interventions of exercise and diet that have shown benefit for both osteoarthritis (OA) and rheumatoid arthritis (RA). For knee OA, over a period of 18 months, exercise plus a healthy diet focused on weight loss showed improvement over baseline values in pain, function, physical performance of a 6-minute walk and stair-climb time, mobility and weight loss.[5]

In other studies on exercise with knee OA, exercise alone showed significant benefit on pain and function with both home-based exercise and walking programs over the course of 3 months.[6] Home strength training for four months showed pain and function benefits, together with improvement in performance, self-efficacy and quality-of-life indicators.[7] Another study compared a program of exercise (weight training plus walking) to exercise plus a weight loss diet for six months. Both groups showed improvement in pain, function, performance, weight loss (more with exercise plus diet), and joint health markers keratan sulfate and inflammatory factor interleukin-1 beta. Most variables showed no significant differences between groups; however, the study was small with only 24 subjects.[8]

Also with knee OA, weight loss diet alone was shown to achieve weight loss, and to improve function and performance of 6-minute walk and stair-climb time as well as improvement in weight, pain, performance, and quality-of-life indicators. Similar effects were achieved in this study with the diet plus electrotherapy (electrical muscle stimulation) for pain relief, but no significant improvements with electrotherapy alone.[9]

For rheumatoid arthritis, a program of bicycle training, exercise circuits, and sport or game, versus standard physical therapy showed greater improvement over two years in general measures of pain and function, and in increased strength and aerobic capacity. No increase in radiographic damage of the large joints was seen, except possibly in patients with considerable baseline damage of the large joints in both groups.[10]

Resistance training plus cycling was added to usual physical therapy to test effects of high intensity exercise on 64 RA patients for 24 weeks versus physical therapy alone. Both groups improved in a measure of tender and swollen joints and overall health. The intensive exercise group's physical function improved significantly, and physical strength improved considerably more than for control group.[11]

Dietary Intervention

A Mediterranean diet has shown benefit for RA at six months. It also has resulted in a decrease in pain and stiffness, and improvement for an index of disability, pain, medication effects, costs of care, and mortality.[12] In another study, for 12 weeks versus control, the Mediterranean diet provided significant improvement in pain, swelling, function and overall health.[13] An anti-inflammatory diet of foods low in arachidonic acid showed significant improvement in RA joint tenderness and stiffness compared to controls, and lower inflammation factors leukotriene b4 and thromboxane, especially when supplemented with fish oil.[14]

Only those patients having had no improvement in the prior two years were selected to participate in this study.

A very low-fat vegan diet showed improvement in RA pain, tenderness, stiffness and function as well as weight loss and C-reactive protein in just four weeks.[15] A 7-10 day fast, followed by a gluten-free vegan diet for three and a half months, then a lactovegetarian diet for nine months showed improvement in RA pain, swelling, grip strength, erythrocyte sedimentation rate, C-reactive protein, white blood cell count, and a health assessment questionnaire score after one month, and again a year later.[16]

Materials and Methods

Subjects

Subjects were drawn from the general public. A group of 18 men and 25 women completed the program with full compliance and adhered to the protocols. All were given diaries and filled out extensive questionnaires listing type of arthritis, symptoms, type of treatment, types of medications, and duration of treatments and outcomes.

Approximately 100 people entered the study, ages 35 to 79 years, with an average age of 61 years. To qualify, participants had to have suffered from arthritis for at least two years and been currently under the care of a physician. Only those patients having had no improvement in the prior two years were selected to participate in this study. Upon examination of entrance questionnaires, it was recognized that many of the participants had unremitting pain symptoms for an average of seven, and as long as 20 years. Anyone who found they could not adhere to the protocol, but would continue to come each week to the meetings, would be used as the control group, and would continue their traditional medical protocols. Subjects presented with both rheumatoid and osteoarthritis and other potentially related disorders – temporomandibular joint disorder, sciatica, spinal stenosis, Ankylosing spondylitis, and herniated discs.

Study Design

This was a lifestyle modification study on the impact of lifestyle and diet on individuals suffering from inflammatory arthritis conditions. The study consisted of instruction on the necessary components of a healthy lifestyle – proper diet, juicing, supplements, detoxification exercise, de-stressing, environmental hygiene, and examination of beliefs and attitudes. Week 1 was an elimination week, with a focus on eliminating dairy, wheat, eggs, sugar, caffeine, artificial sweeteners, refined carbohydrates, cookies, cakes, candies and bread from the diet. Week 2 was a detoxification week with heavy emphasis on juicing multiple times a day with green juices as well as daily exercise in the form of power walking, biking, or deep water running. Week 2 was also the start of the de-stressing phase consisting of journal writing, meditation, taking walks in the park, listening to soothing music, and writing "forgiveness letters" to those who they believed had hurt them, or to those they believed they had hurt in their life. The aim of week 3 was to increase the detoxifying nutrients such as vitamin C, quercetin, vitamin E, glucosamine and chondroitin sulfate, the omega-3 fatty acids, and ashwagandha. Week 4 was focused on increasing detoxification by boosting the consumption of green juices and engaging in journal writing.

Information on the prescribed intervention was given in weekly sessions lasting 2½ hours each, over a period of three weeks from the initial meeting. This executed an intervention of 21 days in duration. 100 persons initially presented at the first meeting; there were a total of 57 individuals who attended every meeting and obtained the information but did not follow the protocol and reported no improvement. This group was used as a control group.

Protocol

Diet

Diet prescribed was an alkalizing anti-inflammatory vegan diet with 75% raw, and 25% lightly cooked foods. It required complete elimination of certain foods, especially pro-inflammatory foods or food preparations, including refined carbohydrates and any wheat, gluten, dairy, meat, poultry and shellfish. No caffeine, alcohol, refined sugar or artificial sweeteners or chemicals such as additives, preservatives, coloring agents or flavorings were allowed; and no carbonated beverages, including sodas and seltzer were included. No conventional table salt, microwaved, deep fried or toasted foods, or nightshade vegetables were permitted.

Allowable were:

- High quality protein from vegetarian sources such as legumes, nuts, seeds and grains – brown rice, Essene bread, millet, amaranth, buckwheat and quinoa. Protein intake ideally was 0.9 g/kg of body weight (40–60g high quality protein for women and 60-80g per men). Fiber intake was at least 35-50 grams.
- Beverages included herbal teas, non-dairy milks – almond, rice, or oat milk, bottled or filtered water, fresh squeezed organic fruit and vegetable juice, coconut milk and coconut water.
- Sweeteners included raw honey, molasses, brown rice syrup, raw palm sugar, natural fruit sweeteners and stevia.
- Oils – grape seed, sesame, extra virgin olive oil, coconut, macadamia and mustard seed oils in moderate amounts. Foods were to be cooked at low temperatures.
- Nine to 12 servings of nutrient-dense fruits and vegetables (preferably organic) per day. Additionally one serving of sea vegetables daily.
- Fruits for anti-inflammation – fresh or frozen berries daily, purple or red grapes, apple, melons, kiwi, citrus, star fruit, papaya, berries and pomegranate.

- Herbs and spices – cayenne, curcumin, basil, rosemary, oregano, thyme, chili peppers, anise, cinnamon, horseradish, wasabi, mustard, dill weed, fennel and spearmint.
- Protein smoothie for breakfast to include berries, 20-25 grams of vegetable protein from powder – pea, rice or hemp, 1000-2000mg vitamin C, 3 oz. of walnuts, rice, almond or oat milk, 1 teaspoon chia powder or seeds, fennel seeds, and 1 teaspoon coconut oil.

Juicing

- 2 juices per day the first week, then increased frequency by one per day – 3 per day the second week, four per day in the third week.
- 16 ounce glasses of a celery, cucumber and apple juice or a watermelon, grapefruit and lemon juice.
- Bok choy, cabbage, cilantro, parsley, kale, collard greens, carrots, beets, beet greens and chard may be added to green juices.
- Dilute green vegetable juices with water.
- Apple seeds removed, citrus can be juiced whole with skin.

Supplements

Can be taken with protein shake, throughout day, or with food for people with sensitivities. Subjects were not required to take all supplements suggested.

Week 1:

- Elimination of all meats and fried foods
- Boswellia, 100 mg
- Cat's claw, 200 mg
- Devil's Claw, 100 mg
- Curcumin, 700 mg with bioperine
- N-acetyl glucosamine, 700 mg
- Ginger, 50 mg
- Vitamin C 3000 mg, divided into three doses throughout the day.

- Chondroitin sulfate, 1200 mg
- MSM, 500 mg
- Hyaluronic acid, 200 mg
- 1 teaspoon coconut oil, can be in cooking

Week 2, add:

- Emulsified cod liver oil (or flaxseed oil), 2 tablespoons on an empty stomach in AM
- Later in day omega-3 essential fatty acids from fish oil, 2000 mg EPA and DHA combined (or flaxseed oil)
- Glass of juice of lemon and grapefruit with quercetin, 500-1000 mg, 4x/day
- Vitamin C to bowel tolerance, 500-1000mg every 3-4 hours
- Curcumin, 1000 mg 5X/day, always with bioperine to increase bioavailability
- Vitamin E, 400 i.u. mixed tocopherols with 100-200 i.u. tocotrienols, 2X/day
- Quercetin, 500 mg, 4X/day
- Cayenne (high heat index) – 50 mg capsule, 2X/day
- Tart cherries, pomegranate, blueberries – fruit juice, concentrate, or extract
- Bromelain, 3x/day w each meal or as directed, or 3 oz. of juiced pineapple core
- Add probiotic formula to breakfast smoothie

Week 3, add:

- 3 oz. of juiced pineapple core blended with ½ teaspoon cinnamon, and added to any liquid to drink throughout the day for anti-inflammation
- Black currant oil at 1000 mg or 1 teaspoon
- 2 oz. of black cumin seed oil

Detoxification

This step is addressed on multiple levels in all parts of the protocol, avoiding pro-inflammatory diet items, use of juicing and supplements to eliminate body toxins, environmental hygiene to eliminate ambient toxins, and the elimination of toxic beliefs, attitude or relationships.

Exercise

Typical prescribed exercise was aerobic exercise such as power walking five days per week, and three days per week resistance exercise. Additional instruction was given for types of exercises that could be done in a seated position for those with significant mobility limitations.

De-stressing

Examples discussed included daily yoga, meditation, tai chi, guided imagery, and mindfulness in nature.

Environmental Hygiene

- De-clutter living space.
- Clean floors and surfaces with safe cleansers – can use hydrogen peroxide or rubbing alcohol.
- Remove indoor pollution sources, including outgassing furniture, carpet, and building materials.
- Use filtered water, and veggie wash or apple vinegar to clean produce.
- Avoid second-hand smoke.
- Acquire house plants or air filter for oxygen purification.

Beliefs and Attitudes for Self Actualization:

Participants were encouraged to examine core values, life purpose, potential for helping others, and to avoid conditioned responses and negative or self-limiting thinking.

Outcome Measures

Of those completing the study, 43 written exit questionnaires and 25 videotaped testimonials were obtained.Questionnaires asked for ratings of changes across nine categories – stiffness, swelling if applicable, pain, range of motion, overall joint improvement, and changes in energy, immune function and sleep. Subjects were to answer whether each category was worse, not changed, slightly improved, improved, or much improved. Participants were asked to write in pertinent information about diagnoses and medications. At the first and last group meetings, measurements were made for blood pressure, and for weight and impedance, from which body fat percentage is calculated, using the Tanita Body Composition Analyzer TBF-300. For video testimonials subjects were asked to identify conditions they had and changes in symptoms over the course of the study.

The study showed that 95% of subjects reported improvement for stiffness, 88% reported improvement for swelling where present, 95% for pain, 89% for range of motion, 86% for muscle use, and 100% reporting overall joint improvement.

Results

As seen by Graphs 1-3, an overwhelming percentage of participants reported improvement in symptoms in all categories. It was shown 95% of subjects reported improvement for stiffness, 88%

reported improvement for swelling where present, 95% for pain, 89% for range of motion, 86% for muscle use, and 100% reporting overall joint improvement. In other categories, 93% of subjects reported improvement in energy, and 65% in immune function. Immune function was measured by asking participants to consider the frequency and severity of their colds and missed sick days compared to previous years after following the protocol for three months. (Data was missing in some questionnaires in that category, possibly due to difficulty in assessing it in the short study duration.) For sleep, 95% of subjects reported improvement. Positive results were noted for subjects with both rheumatoid and osteoarthritis, and other potentially related disorders – temporomandibular joint disorder, sciatica, and Ankylosing spondylitis.

Weight loss and blood pressure were important in this study as secondary outcomes. Tables 1 and 2 show positive results in both areas. Average systolic blood pressure decreased over 10 points, and diastolic pressure over 5 points. Weight loss was analyzed for subjects with a Body Mass Index (BMI) over 27 who could benefit from losing weight. Average weight loss was nearly seven pounds over the three week period, with proportional reduction in BMI. Percentage of body fat shows decrease. These results are important for the topic of this study in that Centers for Disease Control (CDC) data shows that prevalence of arthritis, adjusted for age, increased significantly with BMI for the year's studied.[17] Body fat percentage decreased, but not in proportion to weight loss, and decreased more in men than in women.

The "Exceptional Results" and "Additional Results" section were drawn from videotaped testimonials with clarification from exit survey questionnaires. The exceptional results illustrate the profundity of some of the changes reported, with often long-endured conditions noted.

GRAPH 1*

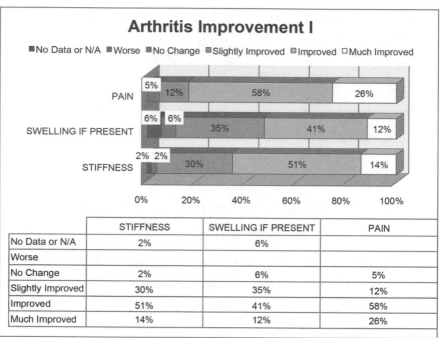

Arthritis Improvement I

■No Data or N/A ■Worse ■No Change ■Slightly Improved ■Improved □Much Improved

	STIFFNESS	SWELLING IF PRESENT	PAIN
No Data or N/A	2%	6%	
Worse			
No Change	2%	6%	5%
Slightly Improved	30%	35%	12%
Improved	51%	41%	58%
Much Improved	14%	12%	26%

GRAPH 2*

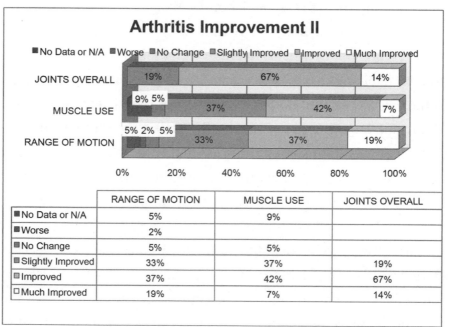

Arthritis Improvement II

■No Data or N/A ■Worse ■No Change ■Slightly Improved ■Improved □Much Improved

	RANGE OF MOTION	MUSCLE USE	JOINTS OVERALL
■No Data or N/A	5%	9%	
■Worse	2%		
■No Change	5%	5%	
■Slightly Improved	33%	37%	19%
■Improved	37%	42%	67%
□Much Improved	19%	7%	14%

Some totals for percentages may not equal exactly 100% due to rounding off of individual figures.

GRAPH 3*

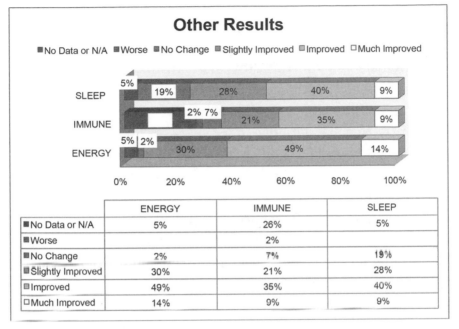

Other Results

■No Data or N/A ■Worse ■No Change ■Slightly Improved ▨Improved □Much Improved

	ENERGY	IMMUNE	SLEEP
■No Data or N/A	5%	26%	5%
■Worse		2%	
■No Change	2%	7%	19%
■Slightly Improved	30%	21%	28%
▨Improved	49%	35%	40%
□Much Improved	14%	9%	9%

Some totals for percentages may not equal exactly 100% due to rounding off of individual figures

Study Group Blood Pressure Results[†]

	AVERAGE SYSTOLIC mmHg			AVERAGE DIASTOLIC mmHg		
	INITIAL	FINAL	CHANGE	INITIAL	FINAL	CHANGE
WOMEN (14)	149.7	138.0	-11.7	86.0	81.1	-4.9
MEN (9)	145.1	137.1	-8.0	92.7	86.4	-6.3
COMBINED (23)	147.9	137.7	-10.2	88.6	83.2	-5.4

†Subjects are those who returned exit questionnaires

Study Group Anthropometrics for Subjects Beginning with BMI > 27[‡]

	AVG WEIGHT IN LBS			AVG BMI			AVG BODY FAT %		
	INITIAL	FINAL	CHANGE	INITIAL	FINAL	CHANGE	INITIAL	FINAL	CHANGE
WOMEN (10)	188.2	182.1	-6.1	30.3	29.6	-0.7	42.6%	41.9%	-0.7%
MEN (6)	228.0	220.0	-8.0	32.0	30.8	-1.2	28.0%	24.0%	-4.0%
COMBINED (16)	203.1	196.3	-6.8	30.9	30.1	-0.8	37.2%	35.2%	-2.0%

‡All subjects returned exit questionnaires

Exceptional Results

- A male age 66, with 33 years arthritis, was freely able to look over his shoulder, which he could not do at all before.
- A female age 73, with 20 years arthritis, previously unable to close her hand, could do so at the end of the study, and eliminated "excruciating" arm pain.
- A male age 64, with five to six years of OA in hips and spine, decided he didn't need recommended surgery, and stopped medication for pain which had decreased from a level of 8-9, to a level 1-2.
- A female, age 69 reported 50-70% improvement for a 6-year-old wrist and thumb injury, 50-60% improvement for a shoulder injury, and 70% improvement for a neck problem of 20 years duration.
- A female, age not given, who could only walk slowly with torn menisci of both knees, by the end of study was walking fast, and walked three miles to the final meeting.
- A male age 53, with affliction of 10 years duration, had improvement in fingers and knees. Previously unable to make a fist, at end of the study he could do so, tightly.
- A female, age 60 was dancing for the first time in years, with much reduced OA pain, more flexibility, and better walking distance.
- A male age 63, with OA for 12 years, had 50% less swelling of his hands, knees, and feet. By the end of the study he was able to do previously difficult deep knee bends, and had just completed a full 2-hour Zumba exercise class.

Discussion

This study of lifestyle intervention on arthritis had highly significant outcomes. Even more remarkable was that the outcomes were obtained in as short a period as 21 days, with follow up of the study at both one and two months showing subjects were improving and sustaining the results. The participants had been under conventional medical care, and without exception had endured poor results, some as long as 20 years. These interventions proved not only effective for arthritis, but also for providing the additional benefits of improved energy, sleep, immunity, lowering of blood pressure, and weight loss. Much of the protocol, especially the supplement portion, has had extensive scientific research showing positive outcomes for arthritic and other conditions. The supplements of the protocol provided the full spectrum of anti-inflammatory nutrients and antioxidants.

Limitation

The study was a relatively small group, with a short duration.

Conclusion

Given the increasing number of individuals afflicted with pro-inflammatory conditions such as arthritis, as well as the thousands of those using non-steroidal anti- inflammatory drugs, prescription and non-prescription, that die each year, this lifestyle and behavior modification protocol should be considered an important alternative approach to conventional treatments.

Arthritis Testimonials

Susan (69 years old)

BEFORE

I've had neck pain for about 30 years. I've also had pain in my lower and middle back. Recently, my hips and my left knee have been stiff, and since I broke my wrist six years ago, I've had arthritis in my wrist and my thumb. I'm on no medications.

AFTER

My pain level has gone down about 50 to 70 percent depending on which part of my body we're talking about. My wrist and my thumb are about 50 percent better. I have had a sports injury in my shoulder for about 20 years and that's probably about 50 – 60 percent better. My neck, which has been a chronic problem for decades, is probably about 70 percent better. So, generally speaking, everything is going in the right direction.

—◄o►—

Jackie (55 years old):

BEFORE

I have arthritis in my knee and lots of pain. It wakes me up at night. It's very difficult to bend my arthritic knee as freely as the other and it has been difficult for me to climb steps. Also, I have mental fog.

How long have you had these symptoms?
Since I fell last March.

Have any medicines helped you?
No.

Have you seen a doctor about any of this?
Yes.

AFTER

What has changed is I'm sleeping better. I have more mobility. Less brain fog, less pain, and more range of motion. With a torn meniscus in my left knee and advanced arthritis, climbing up and down steps was a great challenges; it has not been a challenge this month, which is brand new. My pants and clothes are fitting differently so I see a loss of weight. I'm eliminating on a regular basis. My attitude is better. These are the most notable changes.

How long have you had arthritis?
It was diagnosed last March.

So would you say in the four weeks you've seen a major change?
Yes. I've seen a major change in the last four weeks with the arthritis – the pain and lack of mobility – especially in my left knee.

Audrey (73 years old)

BEFORE

I have a torn meniscus on both knees, and arthritis in both. I'm pre-diabetic, and I have Candida issues.

How long have you had arthritis?
Probably 20 years.

You had it diagnosed?
Yes.

AFTER

I've been doing this program for four weeks, not completely, but getting into it more and more. I have had some healing crises, which I recognize. The major and dramatic thing that has happened is that I wasn't able to close my hands fully. So there's less swelling and I'm able to close my hands. The other dramatic thing is that I have had excruciating pain in my right arm for the last two months, and that pain has left. I have more range of motion, and in spite of a stage IV torn meniscus in my right knee, I'm finding that I'm able to walk and climb stairs better. Another dramatic change is that I have been consistently bloated for the past 10 years, and I've lost half of the bloat already. Interestingly, a fellow around the age of 40 who's an ex-pro soccer player asked me for a date. So I figured I must be looking great because I'm feeling better! And since he wasn't asking my age I wasn't telling.

—◄o►—

John (52 years old)

BEFORE

I have arthritis in both shoulders, both knees and the spine. I was diagnosed maybe a year and a half ago.

Are you on any medications?
No.

AFTER

I was doing okay, and I didn't know I had arthritis because I was involved in another quick protocol with juicing. But I had an accident this time last year, and things went downhill, especially the last six months when I had major pains in my knees. My job is very physical, so I depend on the being mobile. Even sitting down my knees would be in pain. But in the last week, in particular, I have no pain in my knees. I have much more mobility. I can get back to riding my bike and hiking, which I couldn't do before. So I'm feeling much better and more mobile.

◄○►

Nick (77 years old)

BEFORE

I have a mild form of arthritis, but I know my mother died from arthritis. She went through two cancer operations. She survived them without chemo, without radiation; but the arthritis was the thing that really killed her. I took care of her for 13 years, 24/7; and I saw what doctors did. Now my primary doctor wants me to go to see this rheumatologist who used to come to my house every month to take care of my mother, and I don't want to do that. So I want to try this program to see if I can be helped.

AFTER

When I first started this course four weeks ago, I walked down 86th Street, turned off at Third Avenue, and walked across Third Avenue to come down 92nd Street. By the time I reached 92nd Street, I realized the pain that I had in my knees. It took more energy for me to keep from falling forward than it does now. In coming here today, I took the same path. Now I don't have pain like I had then. So I know I'm doing better that way. I just want to say with Gary's help I can see the difference.

Larry (65 years old)

BEFORE

I've had arthritis in my hips for as long as I can remember, about eight years. I didn't realize. When I first felt the pain, I thought I pulled a muscle. It started to really bother me about five years ago, when I started driving private charters– I did not have a doctor at the time. I've been in pain since, and just got a doctor in April because of the pain. They told me they want to replace this hip. I had to stop working full time last year because I couldn't take the pain any more. Some days 400 or 500 miles – lifting suitcases and traveling a lot.

AFTER

I've only been on this a complete three weeks; this is my fourth week going into it. I've learned so much here. I'm in the hospital now because they want to replace this right hip. I thought it was my left hip that needed replacing. The MRI also showed that I have a little arthritis on L3, L4 and L5, and S1 in my spine. But let me say right now before I go any further – the only thing that's going to happen is the right hip. But there will be no surgery for my left hip and my back. I can guarantee it. I'm in PT twice a week. I used to go for an hour and couldn't wait to get out of there. But now I'm in there two and three hours. I walk on the treadmill for 15 minutes; I'm on the horizontal bicycle for 15 minutes; and when I get home I am not that sore. The pain has subsided, I stopped taking pills, I sleep better, and I am a magnificent expression of myself! I thank Gary, Luanne and Dr. Feldman. God bless them all.

—◄o►—

Keith (60 years old)

BEFORE

I have arthritis in both knees, and I never take any medication, only supplements.

How long have you had this?

I would say about seven to eight years.

AFTER

For the four weeks I'm in this program, I've experienced a major improvement in mobility. The heaviness in my knees is practically gone and so is the stiffness. I based my improvement on a simple test. When I first came to the program, I had a little problem getting up the steps. Now I walk up the steps, for the past weeks, with very little pain or stiffness in the knees. One other thing I'm very much surprised about is – I never believed I could have gone without meat for three weeks, and I did. That was a major accomplishment. My health is better. I feel better, and overall I say the program is great.

Robert (53 years old)

BEFORE

I was diagnosed with osteoarthritis in my hands and my knees. So I'm here to make a difference.

How long have you had this?

I notice it has been about eight years now.

AFTER

Arthritis has been a difficult challenge for me. I'm a pretty athletic young man; I do a lot of things. But I haven't been able to do the things I used to do with my kids. What I must say is over this past four weeks I have made a lot of progress. I'm feeling really good about my fingers and my knees. I was actually not able to make a fist with this hand four weeks ago without having difficulty with my fingers. Now this fist is as tight as I can possibly make it, and it's a good feeling. I also had difficulties moving my knees because of swelling and stiffness. But that is reducing. This is a great feeling. This is a great day for me. Within these four weeks, I can feel a great, great improvement – at least 50 percent. I am much more alert, and my bathroom visits have definitely been more frequent. I'm feeling really good.

Andrea (53 years old)

BEFORE

About two months ago I was diagnosed with arthritis in the joints in my fingers; and, of course, you know they want you to take Celebrex. But I don't really want to do that.

How long have you had that pain?

Two months.

AFTER

The decrease in pain is phenomenal and my energy level is really through the roof.

—◄O►—

Rosalind (54 years old)

BEFORE

I have pain in my knees and stiffness in the joints of my fingers, and I'm not taking any medication at this point.

How long have you had that stiffness?

About five years.

AFTER

Over the past four weeks, I've been able to sleep better. I have better elimination. I'm able to walk up and down stairs with no problems. My moods are much better. I don't have the desire for sweets. I can walk past the fast food restaurants and keep going. I have a new relationship with food. I absolutely love vegetables! I'm beginning to learn what food tastes like and it's fabulous. I've had a problem with preparing foods in that I generally have to have meat and seasoning. I don't need that anymore, and I'm so glad to be a part of this program.

Althea (53 years old)

BEFORE

I have been diagnosed with TMJ a little more than a year ago; I also have pain and stiffness in my fingers and sometimes my feet. I have sports-related injuries as well – I tore the ligaments in my left knee, and some in both shoulders. I get acupuncture and I take Chinese herbs and supplements. I haven't taken any drugs.

How long have you had this?

Almost two years.

AFTER

Within just four weeks, I feel a lot of improvement in my flexibility because I'm able to exercise more. I'm also feeling overall more positive and just feeling good. I'm not having any pain in my shoulders, and would typically have more stiffness in my shoulders and in my knees prior to this program.

—◄o►—

Ronald (56 years old)

BEFORE

I have bad arthritis in my both knees. I have to wear braces to support myself. I also have a bad shoulder, my left shoulder. I've had pain in my joints for about ten years, and have been taking supplements for about five years. But I've only been able to slow the progress; I haven't been able to stop it. So I'm hoping to do that here.

AFTER

When I started this program I wasn't able to stand for more than five minutes without my knees buckling. And now four weeks later, I don't mind standing at all. As a matter of fact, I like standing. And I'm walking a lot further and a lot straighter. My pain is about 50 percent less than it was and my flexibility is better. Overall, my lifestyle has improved tremendously. I'm sleeping better, I'm feeling better, and I'm more cognitive in the morning when I wake up. I have Gary to thank for this. Thank you very much, Gary Null.

Donna (55 years old)

BEFORE

I've had arthritis; I'm not exactly sure for how long, but I heard officially approximately five years ago when I had the meniscus removed in both my knees. I lost some weight then, and my knees felt better. I gained the weight back, so my knees don't feel so great now. I've been walking very slowly, and not far distances. I'm walking with, you know, those elasticized things on my knees, and walking is slow. I also have issues with my thumbs – lots of pain using scissors and opening up jars. Things of that nature can be real difficult.

AFTER

Now I am walking far distances, and I credit a lot of it – well all of it to the program; it is fantastic. First of all, I feel incredibly empowered, and I think that's really, really important because you can do anything when you feel empowered. I walked 59 blocks at a brisk pace to get here today, and I feel really good about that.

One year ago I was walking in an airport, and I could hear this person behind me saying, "Gee, I wonder if she drives as slowly as she walks."

Well, three days ago I was walking on a college campus. I was running a little late for a meeting and passed a young woman who I later found out was an undergraduate, so I guess she was between the ages of 19 and 22. And as I passed her she said to me, "Gee, I thought I was walking really quickly, but you're *really* walking, and passing me!" it felt like that comment negated the one from last year. Obviously, my knees feel a lot better. My thumbs, which have been a problem, have improved. They're not perfect yet, but hey, it's only four weeks. So I'm sure they're going to continue to improve. Thank you for everything.

Barbara (60 years old)

BEFORE

I have arthritis in my knees, ankles and lower back, and in my elbows and fingers. I also have high blood pressure.

How long have you had it?

I'd say from '05 and it's terrible. It's terrible because I used to run and do all sorts of athletic things.

AFTER

With the arthritis, as of this time, I don't have any pain. Well, I have a little depending on the weather but that's slight compared to what it used to be. My joints are flexible; I'm able to walk farther and I have no complications as of now. For me, arthritis was for old folks, and I thought I would never get it, but I did. I learned how to deal with it. Recently, however, I went to a party, and I was dancing. I shocked myself because I wasn't able to move that well before. But now I'm able to move. I feel great, and this protocol that Gary put us on works. I don't have meat, so I haven't had meats in quite a while, plus no dairy, and no foods that cause inflammation. I'm doing very well. Plus, the juicing – the green and red juices – fantastic!

◄○►

Maureen (56 years old)

BEFORE

I have knee problems, and problems with my feet and hands with the arthritis. I'm hoping that this will help.

How long have you had the pain?

That was since 2002. I fell and did something to my knees.

AFTER

I've been on this diet just like Gary suggested and my arthritis has definitely improved. I have more flexibility, I can sleep longer, I'm exercising better. I wake up early, brighter and happier. It's helped my mood. It's working for me, and I think that it's going to continue to work, and I'm going to stay with the diet. This is the best I have felt for a long time, and I've lost weight, which is good.

—◄○►—

Jean (60 years old)

BEFORE

I have arthritis in my hips, both my knees and ankles, and in my neck and back. I've had it for about 15 to 20 years, and I'm wearing braces. I'm in a lot of pain.

Are you on any medications?

No. They don't work.

AFTER

Since being on the program for four weeks, I can now sleep on my right side. I couldn't do that before. I've lost about 14 pounds. Everything is feeling a lot better. My fingers used to lock up and were in a lot of pain when they got cold, and they don't hurt as much. I'm going to continue on the program.

Do you feel this program has made a difference?

Oh, yeah. And I can go to the bathroom easier, too.

—◄○►—

Pat (53 years old)

BEFORE

I was recently diagnosed with rheumatoid arthritis, about six months ago after going through Hepatitis C treatment. I have pain in all my joints, and in my feet. Sometimes I can't stand or hold cups.

AFTER

In the last four weeks everything has really changed. My swelling has gone down and my energy has increased; I feel almost normal again. My clarity has improved, and my brain fog is gone. I can think better, and my speech has gotten much better. My speech was very slurred because of the pain. Everything feels better now. My digestion is incredible. It's just amazing.

What would you call the last four weeks?

A growing experience. I've heard of all of this, but I've never really experienced it, and it's pretty incredible. I didn't think this was possible. I thought I was going to be crippled in the next few years, but now I don't believe that.

—◄o►—

Maricela (35 years old)

BEFORE

I was diagnosed with rheumatoid arthritis in 2009. My wrists and knees are swollen, and so is my ankle.

Are you on any medications?

No. I'm not taking medication.

AFTER

It's been three years since I was diagnosed with arthritis. In the last four weeks, my movement has improved and I have more energy and feel better because I can walk. I can move. I couldn't jump before but now I can. It was difficult climbing steps but now I can do this better.

—◄o►—

Tom (57 years old)

BEFORE

I have osteoarthritis in my wrists.

Are you on any medications?

No. I don't take any medicine.

AFTER

In the last four weeks, I've had a 50 percent change in the osteoarthritis in my hands – a 50 percent improvement in the swelling and the pain. Besides that, I've become clearer; I just seem to be getting more things done – the things that I've been procrastinating about. Energy levels have definitely improved, and digestion has been good. After ten years of pain, I've seen improvement in just four weeks. It's pretty amazing actually.

-◄O►-

Wilma (77 years old)

BEFORE

I have several conditions. I have low thyroid and high blood pressure, but I'm here for the arthritis. I've had arthritis for 25 years. I have arthritis in my hands, my neck, shoulder, and knees. The only way I can control my pain is with chondroitin and glucosamine. I didn't take it for a month because I was doing so well; I figured, oh now I can go without it. And within three weeks my hands became claws. I could hardly button anything, and it took me about two to three months to get back to moving my hands. I don't have too much pain right now; but still, my joints are deformed. My neck, though, is really bothering me.

AFTER

What's changed in the last four weeks?

I have a lot more flexibility in my fingers now, and I don't have any pain. I know I'm a work in progress, but I definitely have made improvements. I also have lots of energy; I can walk for hours. I sleep well and have no problems sleeping. My digestion is good and I feel great. The juices I think have helped me a lot, so has getting off of animal protein. The vegetarian diet has definitely improved my well-being.

Lindsey (63 years old)

BEFORE

I was diagnosed with onset osteoarthritis about 12 years ago. Basically, I just have a little stiffness and not really pain so much. I'm here to see how things will work out.

AFTER

I noticed since I've been on the program I've had about a 50 percent decrease in swelling. I had swelling in my hands, and a little bit in my knees and foot. I also had some slight digestive problems. Now, I'm having much better eliminations and I'm feeling better overall. I can do deep knee bends again, which I had trouble with before. So, overall, things are better. Energy is up. As a matter of fact, I took my first Zumba class yesterday, and I made it through the whole class. I didn't think I was going to do it because it was a two-hour class. But it went very well.

—◄o►—

Lou (56 years old)

BEFORE

In February of 2002, my wife and I went to Roseland Ballroom to dance. I started moving down to the floor. It was okay that day, but the next afternoon I was in severe pain. I then went to the hospital, and was diagnosed with osteoarthritis in both knees. The doctor set me up for surgery for one knee, which I had in November of 2002; he schedule me for January 2003 for the other. I asked the doctor if I would get my full range of motion back; he told me that within two weeks it would be like I was in my 20s. Five months after the first knee, I was still pulling myself up the subway staircase with the handrail. So I didn't let him get the other.

Three years later, I fell on a manhole cover and landed on my behind on my tailbone. I went to the osteopath who said that I now was a Level 3 (out of 4) with my arthritis, and "on the other side of the mountain now." I didn't know there was another side of the mountain. I don't like to take pills but pain would come now and then and I would take Aleve, Advil, Tylenol – whatever I could take. And I would also take supplements.

I'm also here for the pain in my back; I had intense pain in my back when I was working at a computer job in 2003.

AFTER

So far, I've lost more than nine and a half pounds in this period of time. I can see my toes! A woman where I live commented that my face had gotten smaller and she also noticed that my gut was gone. I was out last night and my son said, "Stand up. No. Stand up." And I stood up. He said, "Wow! You did that in three weeks?" I said, "Yeah." He said, "I couldn't do that."

I've also got a lot of energy, and can walk. But I mean I can walk faster. I'm aware of it. I still have some swelling, and can feel the knee that was operated on. The pain comes back from time to time; I'm bone to bone because my meniscus is totally gone so that's probably why. But the heaviness in my legs when I used to walk is gone now.

◄O►

Jim (79 years old)

BEFORE

I'm here primarily for my osteoarthritis. It's getting progressively worse and restricting my lifestyle.

Where is it in your body?
Knees primarily, a little in the shoulders.

How long have you had it?
About three years.

Are you on any medications?
No.

AFTER

My primary complaint is arthritis of the knees. I've noticed a drastic improvement in flexibility and resiliency. Whenever I go to the gym, which I do every other day, I can increase or ratchet up the tension. Heretofore, when I would do something like that, I would get jolts of nerve pain and have to back off. But now I can increase gradually without suffering any pain or ill effect. My nutrition has increased dramatically as well. I am primarily on a juice diet. I think carefully about solids – definitely no meats and no fish; strictly veggies and fruits. It's been a remarkable improvement because it has all been upward. I thank Gary and the program for what I've achieved, and I'm looking forward to much more improvement over time.

Section III

A Natural Approach to Arthritis

Introduction

Just as several groups in the medical community suggest erroneously that food has no impact on arthritis and its accompanying pain, we have been told by many within mainstream medicine that nutrients also do not make a difference in treating arthritis. As a point of fact, an extensive body of scientific literature demonstrates that they do.[18,19] The truth is that arthritis patients can benefit significantly from taking vitamins, minerals and other supplements as well as following a whole foods diet abundant in vital nutrients. What follows is a list of the most powerful supplements and foods that have been scientifically proven to aide in the prevention, treatment and reversal of this disease and the painful side effects that accompany it.

> The truth is that arthritis patients can benefit significantly from taking vitamins, minerals and other supplements as well as following a whole foods diet abundant in vital nutrients.

Please also take a look at the charts following these supplements. I have provided guidelines to consider in terms of the priority of these supplements depending on the stage (prevention vs. full-blown symptoms) and type of arthritis that you are dealing with. When in doubt, it is best to consult a nutritionist, naturopathic physician, acupuncturist or other natural health practitioner with knowledge on the subject.

Lastly, it is very important that you consider the quality of these supplements carefully. Natural healthcare professionals often carry a higher standard of product than can be found in health food stores. The majority of the supplements sold in the United States today are manufactured in Chinese factories that are seldom inspected by the

FDA or any other regulatory body.[20] Furthermore, it is important that you as a consumer take time to learn about supplements and their efficacy. For example, vitamin C is more effective when taken with bioflavonoids to ensure maximum assimilation and ideally should be from organically grown whole food sources.

Anti-Arthritis Supplements

Antioxidant Vitamins

Supplementation with antioxidant vitamins directly targets the inflammation and free radical damage that leads to chronic diseases such as arthritis. As a general rule, antioxidant vitamins are extremely helpful in creating health, and are recommended for everyone regardless of current medical conditions. For arthritis in particular, vitamin C is essential for maintaining and repairing bones and cartilage. At least 3,000 mg of vitamin C should be taken throughout the day in divided amounts. Its beneficial effects are amplified when it is taken with glucosamine. Additionally, taking 400 IU of vitamin E and 50,000 IU of vitamin A or beta carotene daily may help to prevent and reduce arthritic pain.

Supplementation with antioxidant vitamins directly targets the inflammation and free radical damage that leads to chronic diseases such as arthritis.

We have provided you with seventeen of the finest nutrients for helping reduce inflammation, swelling, and pain. All of these are backed by voluminous scientific peer-reviewed articles which support their safety and efficacy. However, it's logical that many people would be a bit overwhelmed trying to take this many supplements. The best way to take these supplements is by dividing them in three separate batches. Begin by selecting six supplements and take them for three months. When three months is over, add in the next batch of six and after another three months, add in the remaining five supplements.

It is preferable to start at lower doses of a given nutrient and work your way up slowly. For example, start with 500 mg a day of vitamin C. If you don't experience any gastrointestinal discomfort, then go to 1,000 mg daily after one month. Continue in this fashion until you work your way up to the suggested dosage. It is important to note that not everyone has the same tolerance for nutrients, so if you find you are having a challenge with a given nutrient you can isolate it and take it out of your regimen. It is ideal to take these supplements in the morning mixed in a smoothie with a banana, protein powder and non-dairy milk. This will help buffer any sensitivity to taking these nutrients on an empty stomach and will facilitate their absorption.

Chondroitin Sulfate

This substance works to hold cartilage together at a molecular level, allowing collagen proteins to form tissue. It stimulates repair and helps to limit damage from arthritis. The recommended dose is 1000 mg daily.

Gamma-Linolenic Acid (GLA)

GLA is high in prostaglandins that turn off inflammation and reduce pain. This compound is found in borage, evening primrose and black currant oils. Take 240 mg of GLA daily.

Glucosamine

Glucosamine is a primary nutrient for repairing joint cartilage and tissue damage. Since glucosamine is naturally manufactured by each cell in the body, it is a perfectly safe supplement. The recommended dosage is 1500-2000 mg daily.

Grape Seed Extract

Grape seed extract contains pycnogenol, an antioxidant known to strengthen collagen. Other inflammation-fighting antioxidants found in grape seed extract are proanthocyanidins. Research suggests these compounds benefit arthritis patients.[21] The recommended daily amount is 100 mg.

Niacinamide

This form of vitamin B3 helps both osteoarthritis and rheumatoid arthritis. It is advised to take 150-250 mg of niacinamide before mealtime, three or four times daily. Effects are not immediate, but result in a gradual reduction of symptoms and improved range of motion over time. Niacinamide should not to be confused with niacin.

Omega-3 Fatty Acids

The regular intake of these anti-inflammatory fats is important for everyone. Good sources of omega-3s include fish oil, walnut oil, krill oil and flaxseed oil, as well as chia seeds, salmon and sardines. Research has established the ability of these fats to relieve pain from arthritis.[22,23] The findings of one study which examined the effectiveness of krill oil in treating arthritic patients determined that a relatively modest dose of just 300mg of oil lowered the activity of C-reactive protein – a pro-inflammatory marker by half.[24] The results of another study indicated that supplementation with omega-3 fatty acids from fish oil was especially efficacious in curbing symptoms of arthritis when combined with olive oil.[25] The recommended daily amount is 2000 mg and contains both EPA and DHA. Once again, quality is of the highest importance here in order to ensure that you are avoiding problems associated with fish oils, such as rancidity.

Vitamin B Complex

Take a vitamin B complex containing approximately and 15-50 mg of B1, 50 mg of B2, 100 mg of B5 and 50 mg of vitamin B6. These vitamins regulate nervous system health and enhance the utilization of other nutrients.

Minerals

Minerals play an essential role in joint health. Since the Standard American Diet does not contain adequate quantities of these nutrients, it is no surprise that arthritis is so pervasive.

Adequate supply and absorption of calcium, phosphorus, boron and magnesium are essential for the formation of healthy bones, while zinc and selenium are important for the immune system. Other vital minerals are potassium, copper and manganese. Eating a whole-foods diet rich in raw fruits, vegetables, fresh juices, nuts, seeds, and grains in combination with a multivitamin and mineral supplement can make a positive difference.

We recommend that your daily supplement contain all these minerals but we don't offer dosages since they should be determined by a licensed dietician, or physician, based on multiple individual factors including, weight, age, and exercise levels.

Bromelain

Bromelain is an enzyme derived from pineapple, which studies have found to ameliorate pain and improve physical mobility in arthritis sufferers.[26,27] One study determined that individuals with knee pain given bromelain improved in a dose-dependent fashion; in other words, the more bromelain that was taken, the more improvement patients experienced.[28]

Decursinol

Belonging to the class of chemical compounds known as coumarins, this pain-relieving supplement is derived from a type of root native to Asia. Studies have observed decursinol to protect against oxidative stress and reduce pain and inflammation.[29,30,31] The recommended dosage is 200 mg daily.

Hyaluronic Acid (HA)

This is a naturally occurring substance found in abundance in joint tissues. Hyaluronic acid acts as an important mediator of inflammation and proper tissue formation. Supplementation with 200mg daily is recommended for arthritis sufferers.

Methylsulfonylmethane (MSM)

After water and sodium, MSM – a natural sulfur – is one of the most significant components in the body. Taking 500mg daily helps suppress inflammation related to arthritis and reduce joint pain.

Probiotics

Probiotics refers to the beneficial intestinal bacteria which play a key role in digestion and immunity. Scientific testing on animals links supplementation with these bacteria with a significant reduction in arthritic symptoms.[32,33] Excellent food sources of probiotics are sauerkraut, kimchi, miso, and sour pickles. Probiotic supplements are widely available – take at least 5 billion colony-forming units (CFU) containing multiple strains daily.

Quercetin

Quercetin is a naturally occurring flavonoid found in various foods such as apples, onions and tea. Studies have observed this compound to exhibit immune-boosting, antioxidant activity.[34,35,36] One study found that men dealing with chronic pelvic pain syndrome experienced considerable relief after supplementing with quercetin over the course of one month when compared to the placebo group.[37] This compound works synergistically to amplify the effects of vitamin C. Taking 500mg each day may be helpful.

S-Adenosylmethionine (SAMe)

This is an activated form of methionine that seems to restore white blood cell activity in joint fluid by reversing glutathione depletion. SAMe also serves to protect and rebuild cartilage. A daily dose of 400 mg is considered therapeutic.

Superoxide Dismutase (SOD)

This enzyme should be taken with water on an empty stomach, about a half hour before meals. Supplementation with SOD suppresses pain and inflammation.[38] The benefits of SOD are compounded when it is taken with vitamin E. Taking 2000 mg daily may offer relief to arthritis patients.

Vitamin K

Research implicates this vitamin as a potent anti-inflammatory that helps in the prevention and treatment of arthritis.[39,40] The recommended dose of vitamin K is 2 mg daily.

Anti-Arthritis Herbs and Spices

As with supplements, these herbs and spices should be incorporated into your regimen a few at a time over the course of months. Begin at a low dosage and, if they are well tolerated, work your way up to the recommended dosage.

Aloe Vera

A strong detoxifier of the intestines, aloe vera juice helps cleanse the body of toxins that can cause arthritis. Research implicates the usefulness of this plant taken orally and topically as a natural painkiller and anti-inflammatory for individuals suffering from arthritis.[11,13,13] Drink two fluid ounces of aloe vera juice twice daily on an empty stomach.

Boswellia

The healing properties of the boswellia herb have been recorded in Ayurvedic medical literature for thousands of years. Boswellia works similar to nonsteroidal anti-inflammatory compounds but without the toxic side effects. Studies have demonstrated the efficacy of boswellia in treating arthritis.[44,45,46,47] The recommended dose is 100mg daily.

Cayenne

Derived from cayenne peppers, capsaicin alleviates arthritis pain when applied topically. Research has shown capsaicin cream to help manage pain related to both rheumatoid arthritis and osteoarthritis.[48,49,50] Take 50 mg of high heat intensity cayenne twice daily.

Cat's Claw

A plant native to the Amazon, cat's claw stands out as an anti-arthritis superstar. Studies document the power of this herb to protect against inflammation and aid healing in patients suffering from osteoarthritis.[51,52,53] The suggested dose is 200 mg.

Comfrey

Research shows the success of comfrey in reducing pain and improving mobility in arthritis patients.[54,55,56] One study observed that an ointment formulated from comfrey root extract had a "remarkably potent and clinically relevant effect in reducing acute back pain."[57]

Devil's Claw

A shrub native to southern Africa, devil's claw has been used for centuries as a natural pain-relieving remedy. Today, a wealth of scientific evidence demonstrates the amazing anti-arthritis and analgesic properties of devil's claw.[58,59,60,61] One study which compared the efficacy of devil's claw and the arthritis drug diacerhein in treating osteoarthritis determined that this herb is as effective as, and safer than, pharmaceutical drugs in treating this disease.[62] Take up to 100 mg of this herb daily.

Ginseng

A popular root utilized in Traditional Chinese Medicine, ginseng is increasingly seen in Western medicine as a viable complementary treatment for arthritis and other conditions. Recent findings have shown the promising anti-inflammatory effects of ginseng in animal test subjects with arthritis, and in in-vitro, or "test tube", studies.[63,64] Research also indicates that ginsenosides, the active component of Panax ginseng, limit inflammation in several ways.[65] In addition to acting as an anti-inflammatory, Siberian ginseng has been observed to stimulate the immune system and combat cancer.[66]

Nettles

Nettle leaves display notable arthritis-fighting properties in individuals with osteoarthritis.[67,68] Research indicates that stinging nettle extract inhibits pro-inflammatory factors associated with rheumatoid arthritis.[69] Nettle leaves can be crushed and made into a poultice to decrease rheumatic pain.

Turmeric

The powerful health-boosting properties of turmeric, and its main constituent, curcumin, have been the focus of recent scientific research. Studies conclude that curcumin is an outstanding natural anti-inflammatory that reduces joint pain and stiffness and increases mobility.[70,71,72,73] One study noted the remarkable capacity for curcumin to modulate the metabolism of arachidonic acid – a process that directly contributes to arthritis progression.[74] Combining turmeric with a black pepper, which contains the chemical piperine, increases the bioavailability of curcumin.

White Willow Bark

Sometimes referred to as "nature's aspirin", white willow bark exerts powerful analgesic effects in people suffering from joint pain.[75,76,77] The recommended dose is 400 mg.

The Anti-Arthritis Diet

Vegan Whole Foods

A vegan whole foods diet consists of organic, unprocessed fresh fruits and vegetables as well as whole grains, beans, nuts and seeds. This diet eliminates all meat, poultry, fish, seafood, dairy and eggs. Research has demonstrated that adhering to a plant-based diet helps in the prevention and treatment of numerous ailments, including arthritis.[78,79,80,81] The regular consumption of fruits and vegetables in the form of fresh juices and nutrient-dense powders greatly enhances the body's ability to combat arthritis. Following a whole foods regimen means eating foods that are naturally high in dietary fiber. A high fiber diet is crucial in protecting against degenerative disease and maintaining overall health. Two of my colleagues, Dr. Nuchovich and Jill Barron, advise to "eat the colors of the rainbow," which means include as many colorful fruit and vegetables as possible throughout the week. It is also advisable to "eat locally" whenever possible and when the food is in season in the United States. All of this information is widely available on the internet.

> "Contrary to what most people believe, "organic" does not automatically mean "pesticide-free" or "chemical-free."
>
> – Berkeley University

The Importance of Eating Organic Foods

Because organic foods contain a significantly lower amount of pesticides and chemicals than conventional produce, eating organic foods automatically decreases the possibility of inflammation. Chemicals are toxins, and as such can affect our body's health; this is why it is important to limit the number of chemicals we expose ourselves to through our food and other products. According to the Berkeley University site – "Contrary to what most people believe, "organic" does not automatically mean "pesticide-free" or "chemical-free." In fact, under the laws of most states, organic farmers are allowed to use a wide variety of chemical sprays and powders on their crops. So what does organic mean? It means that these pesticides, if used, must be derived from natural sources, not synthetically manufactured. Also, these pesticides must be applied using equipment that has not been used to apply any synthetic materials for the past three years, and the land being planted cannot have been treated with synthetic materials for that period either. Most organic farmers (and even some conventional farmers, too) employ mechanical and cultural tools to help control pests. These include insect traps, careful crop selection (there are a growing number of disease-resistant varieties), and biological controls (such as predator insects and beneficial microorganisms)."[82]

Below is a list of the most highly sprayed fruits and vegetables. In these cases, it is absolutely essential to purchase organic, if you wish to limit the degenerative effects of these toxins on your body.

Most sprayed:

1. Apples	5. Spinach	9. Potatoes
2. Celery	6. Imported nectarines	10. Domestic blueberries
3. Strawberries	7. Imported grapes	11. Lettuce
4. Peaches	8. Sweet bell peppers	12. Kale/collard greens

The group also lists the "Clean 15," or those that rank lowest in pesticide residues. These are:

1. Onions	6. Sweet peas	11. Cabbage
2. Sweet Corn	7. Mangoes	12. Watermelon
3. Pineapples	8. Eggplant	13. Sweet Potatoes
4. Avocado	9. Domestic cantaloupe	14. Grapefruit
5. Asparagus	10. Kiwi	15. Mushrooms

Alkaline-Forming Foods

The Standard American Diet includes an excess of acid-forming foods such as meat, dairy, refined sugar and flour. Consuming these foods causes the blood pH levels to drop below its ideal range of 7.2 -7.4, and results in an overly acidic state. To compensate for the acid environment, vital alkaline minerals such as calcium and magnesium are leeched from bones and deposited into the bloodstream in a process that weakens bones and joints and promotes arthritis. Research shows a strong connection between an acid pH and poor bone health.[83,84] Furthermore, a lower-than normal pH suppresses the immune system and contributes to the development of many other chronic illnesses. To optimize prevention and healing of chronic diseases such as arthritis, the diet should consist of 80% alkaline-forming foods.

Lower-than normal pH suppresses the immune system and contributes to the development of many other chronic illnesses.

Some common alkaline-forming foods are:

Fruits

apples, apricots, avocados, bananas, berries, currants, dates, figs, grapefruit, grapes, kiwis, lemons, limes, mangoes, melons, nectarines, olives, oranges, papayas, peaches, pears, persimmons, pineapple, quince, raisins, raspberries, strawberries, tangerines and watermelon. (The most alkaline-forming foods are lemons and melons.)

Vegetables

artichoke, asparagus, sprouts, beets and beet greens, bell peppers, broccoli, Brussels sprouts, cabbage, carrots, cauliflower, celery, chard greens, collards, corn, cucumbers, dandelions, eggplant, endive, garlic, ginger, horseradish, kale, lettuce, mushrooms, mustard greens, okra, onions, parsley, potatoes, pumpkin, radishes, spinach, sprouts, squash, tomatoes, watercress, wheatgrass, wild greens and yams. Note – eliminate nightshade vegetables if you are sensitive to them. (See p. 169 for information related to nightshade sensitivity.)

Sea Vegetables

arame, bladderwrack, dulse, hijiki, kelp, kombu, nori, sea palm, wakame

Whole Grains

amaranth, buckwheat, millet, quinoa, teff

Beans/Legumes

lima beans, peas, green beans, soybeans, spouted beans, tempeh (fermented), tofu (fermented)

Nuts and Seeds

almonds, Brazil nuts, chestnuts, coconuts, alfalfa, chia, radish and sesame

N uts, seeds, legumes and beans are also good sources of antioxidants.

Antioxidant-rich Foods

Fruits, vegetables, herbs and spices contain the highest concentrations of these essential, free radical scavenging compounds. Nuts, seeds, legumes and beans are also good sources of antioxidants. Antioxidant content is measured in terms of oxygen radical absorbance capacity (ORAC). A particular food's ORAC is determined through laboratory testing. Many health researchers, scientists and physicians theorize that the higher a food's ORAC score is, the greater its ability to neutralize free radicals and curb inflammation. Research demonstrates the importance of incorporating antioxidant-rich foods into the diet to protect against the progression of arthritis.[85,86,87] A review of data collected in studies from 1948-2011 showed evidence that dietary antioxidants are protective against inflammatory polyarthritis (arthritis that affects five or more joints) and rheumatoid arthritis.[88] Research recently carried out in Japan associated high values of antioxidants in the blood with a lower incidence of arthritis.[89] The findings of another recent study suggest that a higher intake of fresh fruits and vitamin C helps delay the onset of knee osteoarthritis.[90]

Foods Rich in Folic Acid

Research has established a link between folic acid deficiency and rheumatoid arthritis.[91,92] Arthritis patients may benefit from adding folate-rich foods such as asparagus, garbanzo beans, lentils, alfalfa, soy and oats to their diet.

Whole Grains

Grains such as kamut and spelt, as well as grain substitutes like quinoa, millet and amaranth, provide fiber and an array of valuable nutrients that have been shown to stem inflammation and support overall health. Kamut has high levels of potassium, which plays an important part in bone health. Spelt and amaranth are great sources of manganese, a mineral that has been found to reduce pain in osteoarthritis patients.[93,94] Quinoa is notable for containing all the amino acids and has especially high concentrations of lysine, which is essential to the maintenance of bones, tendons and cartilage and the formation of collagen. Research has linked lysine supplementation with improvement in patients with rheumatoid arthritis.[95] Sprouting grains as well as nuts, seeds and beans makes them more digestible and bolsters their nutritional profile considerably.

Healing Foods

FRUITS

Acai Berry

As one of the most antioxidant rich fruits, the acai berry holds great promise as an anti-arthritis food. Studies have observed this berry's exceptional capacity to protect against oxidative stress.[96,97] Research also connects the intake of acai berry juice with significant improvements in patients suffering from joint pain and a limited range of motion.[98]

Acerola

A small fruit native to the American tropics, acerola is an outstanding antioxidant food containing very high levels bioflavonoids and vitamin C. By weight, the vitamin C content of acerola is 10-50 times greater than that of an orange. Studies have observed the ability of this fruit and its chemical components to reduce inflammation. [99,100,101]

Aronia Melanocarpa

Also referred to as the chokeberry, aronia melanocarpa contains high concentrations of polyphenols and other antioxidants that have potent anti-inflammatory characteristics.[102] This berry has been shown to inhibit the expression of altered cell adhesion molecules, which have been discovered to play a role in inflammation.[103] A study published in the *British Journal of Nutrition* determined that chokeberry extract helped control inflammation markers in rats fed a diet high in sugar.[104]

Bilberry

A close relative of the blueberry, the bilberry fruit is gaining popularity as a highly beneficial antioxidant-rich superfood. Bilberries are notable for their high levels of a type of antioxidant known as anthocyanosides. Studies have shown that supplementation with bilberries helps to modulate oxidative stress and inflammation, stabilize tendons, ligaments and cartilage and improve eye health.[105,106,107,108]

Black Currant

Packed with vitamin C and other beneficial phytonutrients, black currants and black currant oil have been observed in studies to exert a favorable effect on inflammatory and oxidative markers.[109,110,111,112]

Blackberries

The dark color of blackberries is indicative of its high antioxidant content made up of compounds such as polyphenols and carotenoids.[113,114,115] In a study published in the *The American Journal of Medical Nutrition,* black raspberries were found to have the highest antioxidant activity out of 1,113 different foods tested.[116] These berries are also a great source of one of the prime anti-inflammatory nutrients, vitamin C.

Blueberry

The various phytochemical constituents of blueberries have been shown to counteract oxidative stress and decrease factors related to inflammation.[117,118,119] Wild blueberries are thought to contain even higher antioxidant content than conventionally grown varieties.[120] A recent study found that rats consuming a diet of 10% freeze-dried blueberry powder had significantly more bone mass than the animals in the control group.[121]

Camu Camu

Native to the Amazon, the vitamin C-rich camu camu fruit offers a range of health benefits.[122,123] The results of a 2008 study published in the *Journal of Cardiology* measured the fruit's potency compared to vitamin C tablets. In their conclusion the authors remarked that "camu camu juice may have powerful anti-oxidative and anti-inflammatory properties, compared to vitamin C tablets containing equivalent vitamin C content."[124]

Cherries

Cherry consumption has been associated with lower levels of uric acid, the compound that contributes to gout and other forms of arthritis.[125] Research published in *The Journal of Nutrition* in 2006 concluded that individuals who consumed Bing cherries over the course of a month showed significant improvement in inflammatory markers.[126] A study of individuals with osteoarthritis taking tart cherry pills for 8 weeks found that more than half of the people experienced improvement in pain and mobility.[127]

Cranberry

Numerous studies have established the considerable anti-inflammatory properties of cranberries.[128,129,130,131] Cranberries are packed with antioxidants including proanthocyanidins, phenols, triterpenoids which give this fruit a high ORAC value.

Elderberry

Long recognized for its immune-boosting properties, research indicates that elderberry has diverse medicinal qualities that may extend to treating arthritis.[132,133] This fruit is high in anthocyanins and several other compounds which have been shown to scavenge free radicals and fight off inflammation.[134]

Guava

An excellent source of powerful antioxidants including lycopene and vitamin C, guava has been reported to have real potential to provide significant relief to patients suffering from inflammatory diseases.[135,136] One guava fruit contains three to four times as much vitamin C as an orange.

Goji Berry

A growing body of research has identified the Himalayan goji berry as a very promising anti-arthritis food due to its high levels of antioxidant activity and impressive array of nutrients.[137,138,139,140,141]

Large quantities of powerful carotenioids such as beta-carotene and zeaxanthin make goji berries an anti-inflammatory superstar.

Kiwi

Numerous studies have established this fruit as an excellent source of antioxidants that work to effectively protect from DNA from oxidative stress.[142,143,144] Kiwi seeds contain alpha-linolenic acid (ALA), a type of omega-3 fatty acid found to help arthritis sufferers.[145]

Mango

The analgesic and antioxidative effects of mango extract have been documented in recent studies.[146,147] Mangoes contain high amounts of a phenol known as mangiferin; research conducted on arthritic mice suggests that this compound inhibits pro-inflammatory proteins and boosts the capacity of anti-inflammatory agents.[148]

Mangosteen

Studies on mangosteen reveal this fruit's impressive anti-arthritis properties.[149,150] Research suggests that mangosteen inhibits the arthritis-causing effects of arachidonic acid.[151] Mangosteen is rich in a class of antioxidants known as xanthones, which are thought to contribute to its anti-inflammatory effects.[152]

Maqui Berry

Native to the Patagonia region of Chile and Argentina, the little-known maqui berry is quickly gaining a reputation as a superfood. Among fruits, the maqui berry is believed to have the highest concentrations of antioxidants, making it a powerful protector against free radical damage and inflammation.[153,154] Maqui berry is rife with a type of anthocyanin called delphinidins, which studies have found to suppress inflammatory signaling associated with rheumatoid arthritis and other conditions.[155,156]

Noni

Preliminary research points to the noni fruit as a highly beneficial food for arthritis sufferers. One study evaluating individuals with osteoarthritis supplementing with noni juice noted reductions in pain and tension levels as well as increased mobility.[157] Noni has extensive antioxidant activity and has been shown to inhibit damaging protein oxidation.[158,159,160] A study from 2010 observed the fruit's ability to lessen pain sensitivity in animal test subjects.[161]

Pomegranate

Pomegranates contain high amounts of polyphenols including ellagic acid, tannins and anthocyanins, which promote healing and decrease inflammation. Studies have demonstrated the capacity of pomegranate to curb inflammatory cell signaling and reduce oxidative stress.[162,163] The findings of recent studies suggest that pomegranate extract improves joint pain in patients with rheumatoid arthritis and modulates inflammation related to osteoarthritis at a molecular level.[164,165]

Oranges

Well known for their immune-boosting phytonutrient content, oranges are a widely available anti-inflammatory food. Research has documented an inverse relationship between orange consumption and rheumatoid arthritis.[166] One study noted significant improvement in rats with adjuvant arthritis that were treated with flavonoids from orange peel.[167] Oranges carry large amounts of a flavonoid known as hesperidin which possesses anti-inflammatory and analgesic properties.[168]

Papaya

The mix of carotenoids, vitamin C, and unique enzymes makes papaya a terrific food for easing inflammation and promoting overall health.[169,170] This fruit has been used for many years to treat arthritis in different parts of the world. Research indicates that papaya modulates inflammation associated with the aging process.[171]

Passion Fruit

Passion fruit offers a sizeable dose of vitamin A, vitamin C, flavonoids, and minerals such as copper, phosphorus and iron. Research has linked passion fruit with the inhibition of pro-inflammatory cytokines and mediators.[172] One study in which passion fruit peel extract was given to females suffering from knee osteoarthritis noted substantial improvement in pain, stiffness as well as physical function when compared to the placebo group, which actually regressed in all categories.[173] Recent analyses have explored the benefits of a compound found in passion fruit called piceatannol, which exhibits potent free radical scavenging activity.[174]

Pineapple

The pineapple contains abundant quantities of bromelain, a type of enzyme that has been shown to protect against a variety of chronic diseases. Research indicates that bromelain suppresses inflammation and moderates joint pain in arthritis patients.[175,176,177,178] One study determined that bromelain inhibited the production of TGF-beta, a protein that – when overproduced – has been associated with the onset of rheumatoid arthritis.[179]

Prune

Prunes contain an abundance of polyphenols and vitamin K, both of which have been found to reduce oxidative stress.[180,181] The high fiber content of prunes aids digestion and detoxification.

Pumpkin

The bright orange color of pumpkin is indicative of its high antioxidant content. Loaded with vitamin A and carotenoids such a lutein and zeaxanthin, pumpkins store various phytonutrients known to limit damage from oxidative stress and suppress inflammation related to rheumatoid arthritis.[182,183,184] One study on rats discovered that the intake of pumpkin seed oil caused a remarkable decrease in markers of arthritis.[185]

Raspberry

Raspberries contain high concentrations of the ellagic acid and anthocyanins, two antioxidants which have been shown to limit inflammation and produce analgesic (pain-relieving) effects.[186,187,188] A recent study carried out by researchers at the University of Rhode Island concluded that the polyphenols in raspberries may protect cartilage and limit the severity of arthritis.[189]

Strawberry

Strawberries contain an abundance of antioxidants including flavonols, anthocyanins and hydroxybenzoic acids which ease inflammation and may be helpful curbing arthritis.[190,191,192,193] Like other fruits and vegetables, it is theorized that the unique blend of micronutrients in strawberries work synergistically to fight inflammation.

Watermelon

Watermelons are packed with several therapeutic phytonutrients including beta carotene, lycopene and vitamin C.[194] Science has demonstrated the ability of these nutrients to reduce oxidative stress and inflammatory markers.[195] Research has connected lower blood plasma levels of lycopene with rheumatoid arthritis.[196] A recent analysis of over 14,000 patients showed an inverse relationship between beta carotene levels in blood and uric acid, which is known to contribute to gout.[197]

VEGETABLES

Alfalfa

Alfalfa is a nutrient-dense food from which arthritis patients may benefit in a number of ways. The high quantities of chlorophyll found in alfalfa relieve joint pain by lowering levels of uric acid. Research suggests that alfalfa inhibits the production of pro-inflammatory cytokines and implicates Biochanin-A – an isoflavone in alfalfa – as an effective anti-inflammatory agent.[198,199]

Arugula

A type of cruciferous vegetable, arugula contains several anti-inflammatory compounds including glucosinolates and vitamin K. Studies have associated low plasma levels of vitamin K with an increased incidence of osteoarthritis.[200,201]

Asparagus

The unique phytonutrients found in asparagus make it a notable anti-inflammatory food. The scientific literature shows the ability of asparagus to boost immunity and reduce inflammation.[202,203] One study associated the tannins, saponins and flavonoids in asparagus to reductions in pain and inflammation in mice.[204]

Barley Grass

Widely touted for its numerous healing properties, barley grass is an excellent food to incorporate into the anti-arthritis diet. This food is abundant in polyphenols and other nutrients such as calcium, vitamin C, and potassium. Studies suggest that barley grass protects cells from oxidative stress and reduces the symptoms of rheumatoid arthritis.[205,206] The chlorophyll in barley grass works as a strong detoxifier and antioxidant, speeding up the healing process.[207]

Broccoli

Studies show that sulforaphane, an organosulfur compound abundant in broccoli, may hold great promise as a treatment for arthritis patients. In a recent analysis published in *Arthritis and Rheumatism*, sulforaphane was found to reduce several markers associated with the onset of rheumatoid arthritis.[208] It was also recently discovered that sulforaphane inhibits the activity of enzymes that cause joint damage in osteoarthritis.[209] Further, broccoli contains a class of compounds known as galactolipids, which studies indicate may be helpful in healing arthritis.[210]

Cabbage

Like cauliflower and other cruciferous vegetables, cabbage contains arthritis fighting indole-3-carbinol (I3C). Recent studies on this vegetable's anti-inflammatory capacity have focused on a compound known as phenethylisothiocyanate, or PEITC. Tests show that PEITC effectively inhibits various forms of inflammation throughout the body.[211,212]

Carrots

The combination of carotenoids, vitamin A, potassium and a multitude of other vital nutrients in carrots and carrot juice can provide important nutritional support for individuals suffering from chronic diseases such as arthritis.[213,214,215]

Cauliflower

Containing a wide variety of micronutrients such as beta carotene, cinnamic acid, quercetin, kaempferol and sulforaphane, cauliflower is a fantastic source of anti-inflammatory nutrition.[216,217] This vegetable also contains indole-3-carbinol (I3C), a compound which is converted to diindolylmethane (DIM) in the body. Research has found DIM to possess anti-arthritis properties.[218]

Celery

Celery has large quantities of potassium, vitamin K and vitamin C, making it a beneficial addition to an anti-arthritis protocol. Celery seed has been used to treat arthritis for centuries, and today, studies have established its medicinal value.[219]

Collard Greens

Large amounts of antioxidant nutrients like beta carotene, vitamin C and manganese as well as anti-inflammatory indole-3-carbinol are found in collard greens. The scientific literature has consistently shown these compounds to decrease oxidative stress and inflammation.[220,221,222]

Fennel

The therapeutic value of fennel has been recognized for centuries. Fennel is composed of numerous anti-inflammatory compounds such as quercetin, rutin and kaempferol glycosides. Research suggests fennel has great potential as a pain-relieving nutraceutical due to its high antioxidant activity.[223,224] Fennel also contains anethole, a constituent that blocks inflammation and suppresses cancer growth.[225]

Kale

Research points to kale as a powerful nutraceutical. This powerhouse of the brassica family is a rich source of antioxidants including vitamin K, vitamin A, carotenoids and flavonoids. Additionally, kale contains metabolites called glucosinolates, which are converted in the body to detoxifying compounds known as isothiocyanates (ITCs). Kale's beneficial chemical constituents have been proven helpful for numerous health conditions, and in fighting off inflammation.[226,227,228,229]

Onion

Rich in flavonoids such as quercetin, onions are an inexpensive addition to any anti-arthritis regimen. Studies confirm the potency of onions in reducing oxidative stress and inflammation.[230,231,232,233] Red onions are generally higher in flavonoids than yellow onions.[234]

Parsley

Parsley contains high levels of antioxidants that may offer significant relief to individuals suffering from inflammation-related disorders. Research has established the ability of parsley and its compounds to counteract oxidative stress and inflammation.[235,236,237]

Radish

Radishes are a good source of free radical-scavenging nutrients such as vitamin C and anthocynanins. These compounds have been found to modulate inflammatory markers and promote healing.[238,239,240]

Spinach

Volumes of evidence implicate spinach as a phytonutrient powerhouse that can aid arthritis sufferers in many ways. Spinach is an excellent source of vitamin K, a nutrient that is critical to bone health.[241,242] Studies confirm that the antioxidants contained in spinach leaves have impressive anti-inflammatory capabilities.[243,244] It also provides significant amounts of vitamin D, which is necessary for strong bones.[245]

More Healing Foods

Chia Seed

Chia seeds are a superior source of omega-3 fatty acids such as alpha-linolenic acid (ALA). Studies reflect the capacity of omega-3s to fight arthritis-related inflammation.[246,247] Researchers have found that compounds found in these fats known as resolvins are remarkably effective at reducing pain associated with arthritis.[248]

Chlorella

Chlorella is a type of algae packed with a diverse set of detoxifying agents, vitamins, minerals and amino acids. Chlorella has been observed in studies to reduce oxidative DNA damage and various forms of inflammation.[249,250,251] The scientific evidence points to chlorella as a helpful nutraceutical in the prevention and treatment of arthritis.[252]

Coconut Oil

A natural form of saturated fat, coconut oil supports cardiovascular health and boosts immunity. Studies indicate that virgin coconut oil has anti-inflammatory and analgesic properties as well.[253,254] Like all healthy fats, it should be taken in moderation.

Flax Seed

The high levels omega-3 fatty acids in flaxseeds help to strengthen joints by producing inflammation-fighting molecules called series 1 and series 3 prostaglandins.[255,256,257] An important type of omega-3 present in flaxseeds is alpha-linolenic acid, which is known to support bone health.[258] A recent meta-analysis by researchers in Canada determined that supplementation with omega-3s may be an "attractive adjunctive treatment for joint pain associated with rheumatoid arthritis" and other disorders.[259]

Garlic

Garlic offers many health benefits and individuals looking to prevent and treat chronic diseases such as arthritis are advised

Garlic offers many health benefits and individuals looking to prevent and treat chronic diseases such as arthritis are advised to incorporate this superfood into their diet.

to incorporate this superfood into their diet. Garlic is abundant in anti-inflammatory sulfur compounds such as diallyl sulfide (DAS) and thiacremonone, which have been shown to fight arthritis.[260,261,262] One study on the effects of garlic supplementation in rheumatoid arthritis patients determined that 86.5% of all patients experienced a good or partial response.[263] Consuming raw garlic provides the most benefit.

Ginger Root

The benefits of ginger on arthritis patients have been well documented for decades.[264,265,266] A group of powerful antioxidants unique to ginger, called gingerols, are a relative of capsaicin and piperine, the compounds that are responsible for the respective spiciness of chili peppers and black pepper. Research using these chemical components to treat rheumatoid arthritis in animal test subjects has yielded highly positive results.[267]

Green Tea

Widely hailed for its medicinal qualities, green tea possesses numerous compounds that promote joint health and mitigate the impact of various types of arthritis.[268,269,270,271]. One principal antioxidant found in green tea is a type of catechin called epigallocatechin-3-gallate (EGCG). Studies have observed EGCG to suppress osteoclast formation associated with rheumatoid arthritis.[272] Only use decaffeinated.

Spirulina

Also known as blue-green algae, spirulina holds great promise as a natural means of curbing arthritis and promoting healing throughout the body.[273,274] In tests on mice, spirulina was found to significantly decrease inflammation related to arthritis.[275] The authors of one study observed that mice with arthritis given oral doses of spirulina recovered to "near normal conditions."[276]

Foods to Avoid

High-Acid Foods

The consumption of high-acid foods such as refined sugar and flour, dairy, meat, seafood, soft drinks and alcohol is strongly associated with the symptoms of arthritis.[277,278,279,280,281] Pork is especially deleterious, whether it is in the form of ham, bacon, or foods cooked in lard. The intake of coffee is also associated with this disease.[282] In addition to their damaging sugar content, carbonated soft drinks contain high amounts of phosphates, which alter the mineral balance in the body.[283] To promote and optimize healing, these pro-inflammatory staples of the Standard American Diet should be removed. Note – if you are going to consume animal flesh, modest amounts of wild and organic fish (not farm-raised) are best.

Processed and Artificial Foods

Deep-fried, overcooked and processed foods should not be eaten as they are often toxic and nutritionally deficient. It is also important to stay away from artificial foods including trans fats (partially hydrogenated oils) and all synthetic sweeteners including Splenda, NutraSweet and Equal. Other substances to avoid are artificial colors, food additives and preservatives. Genetically Modified (GM) foods are increasingly prevalent in our food supply in products containing corn, soy, and canola oil. A growing body of evidence links genetically-engineered crops with a multitude of health complications including arthritis.[284]

Smoking

Strong scientific evidence connects smoking with the progression of arthritis.[285,286,287,288] Dropping this habit is crucial to preventing and treating this disease.

Conventional Medications

While arthritis medications such as non-steroidal anti-inflammatory drugs (NSAIDs) may appear helpful initially, in the long term they are damaging to overall health.

Nightshade Vegetables

A minority of arthritis patients benefit from avoiding nightshade – vegetables including tomatoes, potatoes, eggplant, bell peppers, paprika, and cayenne peppers. Nightshades contain a substance called alkaloids, which can increase inflammation and compromise joint function. You can find out if nightshades exacerbate joint pain by eliminating them from the diet for 30 days and then eating all of them in one day. If you do not feel any worse after challenging yourself in this way, then you do not need to worry. If symptoms become more pronounced, avoid these foods.

Other Beneficial Additions to the Anti-arthritis Lifestyle

Pure Water

Many arthritis patients suffer from dehydration without knowing it. Water is necessary for joints to function properly and staying hydrated throughout the day is vitally important. Water purity is a large consideration since many local water systems in the United States are contaminated by toxins including bacteria, parasites, heavy metals and chemicals. It is therefore imperative to use a high-quality filtration system to minimize hazardous materials from your drinking supply.

> Water is necessary for joints to function properly and staying hydrated throughout the day is vitally important.

Exercise

Research clearly shows that regular exercise is indispensable for arthritis patients.[289,290,291,292] Engaging in both aerobic and anaerobic exercise is crucial for restoring mobility and function as well as maintaining and building muscle mass, as are exercises that promote flexibility. It is important to note that low-impact exercises are best for joint health and that people should not push themselves beyond their limits. Not only should exercise be appropriate for your level of fitness, but also for your body mass. Stress your muscles in a reasonable fashion, but pain is a warning sign to slow down. People should also wait until they are comfortable enough to engage in activities. If you are considering taking up a new sport or trying a new piece of equipment at the gym, please get guidance. For new sports, it is advised – unless you are in excellent physical condition – that you practice the movements of the exercise that you anticipate doing prior to actually doing the sport; this will help you determine your body's readiness for that particular sport. If there is any pain or tightness when performing these movements, engage in alternative exercises first that can help you prepare your body for the new sport. In the gym, always get help on new equipment, and make your first workout on the new equipment slightly lighter than you might want to just to see how your body responds to the new activity. Have no doubt that the wrong kind of exercise can worsen arthritic conditions.

Additionally, you will want to choose exercises that you enjoy, and that recreate the mind. One of the most significant benefits of exercise is that it gives your mind a break from its constant chatter. Both endurance and resistance exercises are encouraged, and sweating is a fantastic detoxifier. Moderate-intensity, low-impact endurance exercise has been shown to be ideal for people suffering from arthritis. Moderate-intensity exercise, where you keep your heart rate at 60 - 70% of its maximum, is ideal also for fat burning, especially for longer workouts of 45 minutes or more. Resistance exercises like weight lifting and yoga are essential for increasing muscular strength, which aids in structural stability and joint health, and for maintaining good bone density, which is especially crucial in avoiding osteoporosis.

Walking is excellent for the total body and a good way for the novice to begin. It can improve circulation in the hands, knees, shoulders and fingers, areas commonly affected by arthritis. Engaging in swimming and water walking offers a good workout without causing excessive stress or pain in the joints. I also recommend elliptical machines for arthritis sufferers, the ROM machine is one example of this. These machines result in less strain on the joints overall, and are more supportive if you are carrying extra weight. Mini trampolines called "rebounders" are excellent for building strength and for improving fitness levels while assisting with detoxification – the gravitational force helps to clean the lymph system. It is possible to run in place on these trampolines and get your heart rate up; however, it is a much lower impact exercise than running on pavement. Rebounders come with stabilizing bars for people with balance issues.

Yoga is another beneficial practice for people of all ages. Slow stretches lubricate joints and increase flexibility while special breathing techniques expel toxins in the joints and muscles, and decrease mental and emotional stress. There are many different types of yoga, including therapeutic yoga, and they can vary greatly. It is best to speak to a professional prior to deciding which classes are best for your current level of physical conditioning. Some yoga styles can be an extremely rigorous and inappropriate for beginners, and movements must be done properly to avoid injury. If you are a beginner or suffering from physical challenges, let your teacher know prior to class.

Yoga is another beneficial practice for people of all ages.

There are also numerous techniques that promote proper musculoskeletal (and therefore joint) alignment that fall under the category of exercise rather than therapy. Some examples of these movement exercises are Pilates, Muscle Activation Technique (M.A.T.), Yamuna Body Rolling, Gyrotonic® and Gyrokinesis®, and Alexander Technique. These exercises increase our body awareness, and promote improved muscular performance because they work to correct postural alignment and improve body mechanics, among other things. The mistake that some people make in evaluating and treating muscular pain is that they work to rehabilitate the muscles that are in pain (typically the ones that are overcompensating) without addressing the core structural problem that caused the imbalance in the first place. When we have a structural imbalance – whether from birth, accident, or chronic repetitive movements – some muscles become weak and others work harder to overcompensate; this can cause tightness and chronic pain. If the core structural problem is not addressed, and muscles are stimulated into inappropriate action, pain as well as joint stress will occur. It is wise, then, whether you are aiming to prevent or alleviate arthritis that you attend to body mechanics in addition to exercises that improve lung and heart function.

If your current physical condition does not permit you to be up and around, then consider alternative forms of exercise. There are DVDs available for people who cannot move their bodies; "Sit and Be Fit" is just one of the videos that will get you started on the path to movement. There are also "chair" yoga videos that can be used for multiple benefits, as well as whole body vibration technology.

Lifestyle Practices that Promote Emotional and Physical Well-being

The average citizen, let alone a person suffering from arthritis, is probably not aware of the extensive amount of studies (totaling into the thousands) that have established the direct relationship between what we think about and what manifests in our body, otherwise known as psychoneuroimmunology. As a result, the majority of arthritis sufferers don't reap the benefits of the numerous lifestyle practices which have been shown to be safe and effective at improving quality of life. These therapies include

Practices such as Tai Chi, yoga, and meditation have proven to provide numerous physical, mental and emotional benefits.

energy balancing methods such as Chi Gong, an ancient Chinese technique of channeling energy into an area of the body to open up energy pathways, allowing healing to occur.

Practices such as Tai Chi, yoga, and meditation have proven to provide numerous physical, mental and emotional benefits. Other physical therapies like hydrotherapy – the alternating use of cold and hot water on the body – have helped individuals improve circulation and ease the musculature since the times of antiquity in places like Mesopotamia and Greece. Relaxation practices like deep breathing, mindfulness meditation and listening to soothing music, are all underutilized in our society, but are enormously helpful for diminishing stress and aiding in rebalancing hormones. Further, it is my experience that by focusing upon positive outcomes with positive thoughts, we create what I call a positive epigenetic hormonal biochemical healing process that allows us to limit the impact of genetic predispositions and positively influence and strengthen our DNA. Because every thought manifests instantly as a physical reality, our hormones, blood pressure, digestion and neurological activity all respond instantaneously in a positive or negative sense to what you are thinking. Hence, when we say that stress kills, what we mean is that stressful thoughts raise cortisol and other stress-related hormones, which creates a "fight or flight" chemical response in our bodies that, when ongoing, can lead to chronic disease and early death.

These practices, along with an anti-inflammatory diet, nurturing supplements, and appropriate exercises and physical therapies form a holistic protocol that is and has been the cornerstone of success with our program.

Alternative Arthritis Therapies Effective in the Treatment of Arthritis

Acupressure

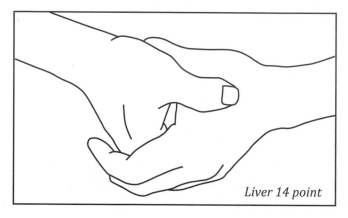

Liver 14 point

Acupressure, which is derived from Acupuncture, is the practice of applying physical pressure to specific meridian points for the purposes of either decreasing or stimulating activity in a particular area of the body. Acupressure can be extremely helpful in alleviating pain from arthritis. In particular, stimulating the point known as "Liver 14" (L14) in the dam between the thumb and the forefinger several times a day can be helpful in reducing pain in the body.

Acupuncture (Traditional Chinese Medicine, including Chinese Herbs)

According to Traditional Chinese Medicine (TCM), acupuncture helps rebalance the body's vital energy, or qi, by inserting small

Acupuncture has proven exceedingly helpful in relieving and mitigating inflammation and pain, including the pain related to arthritic conditions.

needles into the skin at different points. This practice has been used by countless people throughout the world to help reduce the pain and suffering of arthritis, and as an ongoing measure in the prevention and eradication of stagnation that causes, and prevents the healing of, arthritis. There are two treatment paths in TCM related to arthritis – one for "deficiencies" like osteoarthritis, which uses nourishing herbs and treatments that bring energy to the area, and one for "excesses" as in the case of rheumatoid arthritis (excessive heat and dampness), which focuses on using cooling herbs and draining treatments. Acupuncture has proven exceedingly helpful in relieving and mitigating inflammation and pain, including the pain related to arthritic conditions. It also provides excellent support for other challenging causes and symptoms such as erratic sleep, excessive stress and anxiety, and emotional imbalances. A comprehensive study by the National Institutes of Health determined that acupuncture is an effective complement to conventional medicine in treating osteoarthritis.[293] A four-year study by researchers at the University of Maryland School of Medicine published in the *Annals of Internal Medicine* showed that acupuncture provided significant relief to osteoarthritis patients experiencing moderate to severe pain even though they were taking pain medication.[294]

Chelation Therapy

Chelation is an adjunctive therapy that rids the body of toxic heavy metals and plaque. By improving overall circulatory functioning and lessening free radical damage, chelation can reduce arthritic symptoms. This therapy is particularly good for alleviating the crippling effects of rheumatoid arthritis. Scientists hypothesize that the chelation drug EDTA has similar chemical properties to penicillamine, a drug rheumatologists use to treat the disease.

Chiropractic

Chiropractic care is a gentle, safe and noninvasive way for patients to relieve the symptoms of osteoarthritis. During treatment, spinal adjustments are given to release nerve pressure; this allows nerve energy to flow properly. Circulation increases to the joints, enabling them to function better and to heal. This form of therapy increases range of motion, alleviates pain and lengthens the spine, allowing the person to stand straighter and appear taller. Also, by encouraging proper posture, chiropractic treatments minimize pressure on the joints.

Colon Therapy

Many arthritic patients have constipation from an accumulation of toxins in the colon and the body. They suffer autotoxic reactions, including inflammation, as the body responds to the toxins. Autotoxins exacerbate any disease, including arthritis.

Colonic irrigation, or colon hydrotherapy, opens the digestive tract and thoroughly removes accumulated wastes, eliminating toxic substances and harmful bacteria. A series of treatments leaves a person feeling lighter, cleaner and more alive. When colon therapy is combined with an improved diet and supplementation, proper balance is restored. As a result, mobility increases and arthritis may even disappear.

Homeopathy

Homeopathic remedies for arthritis, like those for other ailments, are keyed to very specific conditions:

Rhus Toxicodendron

Used for pain that worsens at night and in the morning upon awakening. Pain is worse in cold, damp weather and before a storm. The person feels better with heat and motion.

Rhododendron

For joint pains that feel worse in the morning, before a storm or weather change, and in heavy winds. Symptoms are alleviated with heat and motion.

Calcaea Carbonica

For pain that is worse in cold, damp weather when there is exertion and motion, and when the limb is hanging downward.

Aconitum Napellus

For pain and inflammation, especially when the skin is hot.

Magnets

Every cell in our body is magnetized. Imbalances occur when we are affected by trauma, disease, or infection, and hundreds of studies show that magnet therapy can be a powerful rebalancing modality. For example, using fixed magnets placed at the base of patients' heads, Dr. William Philpott, M.D., helped remedy numerous cases of depression. I've personally interviewed dozens of his patients who have confirmed the efficacy of this therapy. Additionally, other scientists and physicians are now using electromagnetic pulses with even more beneficial results.

Alternative Diagnostic Procedures in Support of a Healthy Vegetarian Lifestyle

Allergy Testing for Problem Foods

Since allergic responses to foods are a leading cause of inflammation and, therefore, arthritis, skin and blood allergy tests administered by a complementary physician can be valuable for revealing problem foods and chemicals. Completely eliminate foods that you are highly sensitive to, at least for a while. Later, some of these foods can be returned, potentially, to the diet. Foods that cause less of a reaction can be eaten infrequently on a rotation diet, in which the same food is not eaten more than once every four to seven days. For example, if wheat is eaten on Monday, it is not eaten again until Friday, at the earliest.

Environmental Considerations

- Sleep in darkness
- Control your environment:
  - Make sure not to bring foods in the home that are not supportive of your goal
  - Eat some healthy food prior to going to parties; it will help you to resist overeating foods that are not supportive
  - Enroll immediate family and friends in supporting your program
  - Have set meal times, and do not snack in front of TV
  - Use handkerchiefs to open doors, hand sanitizer after being out in public, etc.
- Create good ergonomics in home and at work. If you work on a computer regularly, make sure that you provide proper support for all areas of the body that require it, including proper desk height, foot support, and padding for the wrist when using a mouse.
- De-clutter your home
- Shield from EMFs
- Limit your use of microwave ovens; or get rid of it completely
- Limit your use of cell phone; always use hands-free devices
- Household tips:
  - Clean cooking and eating surfaces and door knobs with Hydrogen peroxide
  - Use natural products for all other cleaning needs
  - Deal with mold remediation if necessary
  - Clean A/C ducts and vents annually, if you use A/C
  - Place toothbrush in hydrogen peroxide after brushing to kill germs

Bibliography, Section II and III

1   Centers for Disease Control. Available at : http://www.cdc.gov/ mmwr/preview/mmwrhtml/mm5939a1.htm?s_cid=mm5939a1_w accessed 3/25/12.

2   Arthritis Prevalence and Activity Limitations -- United States, 1990. *Centers for Disease Control and Prevention.* http://www.cdc.gov/ mmwr/preview/mmwrhtml/00031480.htm accessed 10/5/12.

3   Centers for Disease Control. Available at : http://www.ncbi.nlm.nih. gov/pubmed/16385518 accessed 3/25/12.

4   Singh G. Recent considerations in nonsteroidal anti-inflammatory drug gastropathy. *Am J Med.* 1998; 105:31S–38S.

5   Focht BC, Rejeski WJ, Ambrosius WT, Katula JA, Messier SP. Exercise, self-efficacy, and mobility performance in overweight and obese older adults with knee osteoarthritis. *Arthritis Rheum.* 2005;53:659–65.

6   Evcik D, Sonel B. Effectiveness of a home based exercise therapy and walking program on osteoarthritis of the knee. *Rheumatol Int.* 2002;22:103–106.

7   Baker KR, Nelson ME, Felson DT, Layne JE, Sarno R, Roubenoff R. The efficacy of home based progressive strength training in older adults with knee osteoarthritis : a randomized controlled trial. *J Rheumatol.* 2001;28:1655–65.

8   Messier SP, Loeser RF, Mitchell MN, et al. Exercise and weight loss in obese older adults with knee osteoarthritis : a preliminary study. *J Am Geriatr Soc.* 2000;48:1062–1072.

9   Huang MH, Chen CH, Chen TW, Weng MC, Wang WT, Wang YL. The effects of weight reduction on the rehabilitation of patients with knee osteoarthritis and obesity. *Arthritis Care Res.* 2000;13(6):398–405.

10 Jong Z, Munneke M, Zwinderman AH, Kroon HM, Jansen A, Ronday KH, et al. Is a long-term high-intensity exercise program effective and safe in patients with rheumatoid arthritis? Results of a randomized controlled trial. *Arthritis Rheum.* 2003;48:2415–2424. doi : 10.1002/art.11216.

11 Van Den Ende CHM, Hazes JMW, Le Cessie S, et al. Comparison of high and low intensity training in well controlled rheumatoid arthritis. Results of a randomised clinical trial. *Annals of the Rheumatic Diseases.* 1996; 55(11):798–805.

12 McKellar G, Morrison E, McEntegart A, Hampson R, Tierney A, Macklec G, et al. A pilot study of a Mediterranean-type diet intervention in female patients with rheumatoid arthritis living in areas of social deprivation in Glasgow. *Ann Rheum Dis.* 2007;66(9):1239–1243.

13 Skoldstam L, Hagfors L, Johansson G. An experimental study of a Mediterranean diet intervention for patients with rheumatoid arthritis. *Ann Rheum Dis.* 2003;62:208–214. doi : 10.1136/ard.62.3.208.

14 Adam O, Beringer C, Kless T. et al. Anti-inflammatory effects of a low arachidonic acid diet and fish oil in patients with rheumatoid arthritis. *Rheumatol Int.* 2003;23:27–36.

15 McDougall J, Bruce B, Spiller G, Westerdahl J, McDougall M.Effects of a very low-fat, vegan diet in subjects with rheumatoid arthritis. *J Altern Complement Med.* 2002 Feb;8(1):71-5.

16 Kjeldsen-Kragh J, Haugen M, Borchgrevink CF, et al. Controlled trial of fasting and one-year vegetarian diet in rheumatoid arthritis. *Lancet.* 1991;338:899–902.

17 Cheng, YJ, et al. Prevalence of Doctor-Diagnosed Arthritis and Arthritis-Attributable Activity Limitation – United States, 2007— 2009. *Centers for Disease Control and Prevention.* http://www.cdc.gov/mmwr/preview/mmwrhtml/mm5939a1.htm; accessed 10/5/12.

18 Adam O, Beringer C, Kless T. et al. Anti-inflammatory effects of a low arachidonic acid diet and fish oil in patients with rheumatoid arthritis. *Rheumatol Int.* 2003;23:27–36.

19 McKellar G, Morrison E, McEntegart A, Hampson R, Tierney A, Macklec G, et al. A pilot study of a Mediterranean-type diet intervention in female patients with rheumatoid arthritis living in areas of social deprivation in Glasgow. *Ann Rheum Dis.* 2007;66(9):1239–1243.

20 Harris, Gardiner. "Study Finds Supplements Contain Contaminants."*New York Times* 25 May 2010 : n. pag. A15 nytimes. com. Web. 6 Oct. 2012.

21 Park, MK, et al. "Grape seed proanthocyanidin extract (GSPE) differentially regulates Foxp3(+) regulatory and IL-17(+) pathogenic T cell in autoimmune arthritis." *Immunology Letters* 135, no. 1-2 (2011) : 50-8. http://www.ncbi.nlm.nih.gov/pubmed/20933009 (accessed April 9, 2012).

22 Galarraga B, Ho M, Youssef HM, Hill A, McMahon H, Hall C, Ogston S, Nuki G, Belch JJ. Cod liver oil (n-3 fatty acids) as an non-steroidal anti-inflammatory drug sparing agent in rheumatoid arthritis. *Rheumatology* (Oxford). 2008 May;47(5):665-9.

23 Goldberg RJ, Katz J. A meta-analysis of the analgesic effects of omega-3 polyunsaturated fatty acid supplementation for inflammatory joint pain. *Pain.* 2007 May;129(1-2):210-23.

24 Deutsch L. Evaluation of the effect of Neptune Krill Oil on chronic inflammation and arthritic symptoms. *J Am Coll Nutr.* 2007 Feb;26(1):39-48.

25 Berbert, AA, et al. "Supplementation of fish oil and olive oil in patients with rheumatoid arthritis." *Nutrition* 21, no. 2 (2005) : 131-6.

26 Klein G, Kullich W. Short-term treatment of painful osteoarthritis of the knee with oral enzymes. A randomized, double-blind study versus diclofenac. *Clin Drug Invest.* 2000;19(1):15-23.

27 Desser, L, et al. "Oral therapy with proteolytic enzymes decreases excessive TGF-beta levels in human blood." *Cancer Chemotherapy and Pharmacology* 47 (2001) : S10-15.

28 Walker, AF, et al. "Bromelain reduces mild acute knee pain and improves well-being in a dose-dependent fashion in an open study of otherwise healthy adults." *Phytomedicine* 9, no. 8 (2002) : 681-6.

29 Kang, SY, and YC Kim. "Decursinol and decursin protect primary cultured rat cortical cells from glutamate-induced neurotoxicit." *The Journal of Pharmacy and Pharmacology* 59, no. 6 (2007) : 863-70. http://www.ncbi.nlm.nih.gov/pubmed/17637179 (accessed May 7, 2012).

30 Kim, JH, et al. "Decursin inhibits induction of inflammatory mediators by blocking nuclear factor-kappaB activation in macrophages." *Molecular Pharmacology* 69, no. 6 (2006) : 1783-90. http://www.ncbi.nlm.nih.gov/pubmed?term=Decursin%20inhibits%20induction%20of%20inflammatory%20mediators%20by%20blocking%20nuclear%20factor-kappaB%20activation%20in%20macrophages. (accessed May 13, 2012).

[31]   Choi, SS,et al. "Antinociceptive mechanisms of orally administered decursinol in the mouse." *Life Sciences* 73, no. 4 (2003) : 471-85. http://www.bronsonvitamins.com/decursinol-50-for-pain-and-more (accessed May 8, 2012).

[32]   Nowak , B, et al. "Lactobacillus rhamnosus Exopolysaccharide Ameliorates Arthritis Induced by the Systemic Injection of Collagen and Lipopolysaccharide in DBA/1 Mice." *Arch Immunol Ther Exp* (Warsz) Epub April 8 (2012). http://www.ncbi.nlm.nih.gov/pubmed/22484803 (accessed May 13, 2012).

[33]   So, JS, et al. "Lactobacillus casei enhances type II collagen/glucosamine-mediated suppression of inflammatory responses in experimental osteoarthritis." *Life Sciences* 88, no. 7-8 (2011) : 358-66. http://www.ncbi.nlm.nih.gov/pubmed/21167838 (accessed May 7, 2012).

[34]   Lamson DW, Brignall MS. Antioxidant and cancer III : quercetin. Altern Med Rev 2000;5:196-208.

[35]   Guardia T, Rotelli AE, Juarez AO, Pelzer LE. Anti-inflammatory properties of plant flavonoids. Effects of rutin, quercetin, and hesperidin on adjuvant arthritis in rat. *Farmaco.* 2001;56(9):683-687.

[36]   Ruiz PA, Braune A, Holzlwimmer G, Quintanilla-Fend L, Haller D. Quercetin inhibits TNF-induced NF-kappaB transcription factor recruitment to proinflammatory gene promoters in murine intestinal epithelial cells. *J Nutr.* 2007 May;137(5):1208-15.

[37]   Shoskes D, et al. Quercetin in men with category III chronic prostatitis : a preliminary prospective, double-blind, placebo-controlled trial. *Urology* 1999;54:960-3.

[38]   Kelkka, T, et al. "Superoxide dismutase 3 limits collagen-induced arthritis in the absence of phagocyte oxidative burst." *Mediators of Inflammation* Epub March 5 (2012) : . http://www.ncbi.nlm.nih.gov/pubmed/22529530 (accessed May 1, 2012).

[39]   Oka, H. "Association of low dietary vitamin K intake with radiographic knee osteoarthritis in the Japanese elderly population : dietary survey in a population-based cohort of the ROAD study." *Journal of Orthopaedic Science* 14, no. 6 (2009) : 687-92. http://www.ncbi.nlm.nih.gov/pubmed/19997813 (accessed April 10, 2012).

[40] Neogi T, Booth SL, Zhang YQ, et al. Low vitamin K status is associated with osteoarthritis in the hand and knee. *Arthritis Rheum* 2006;54:1255–61.

[41] Cowan, D. "Oral Aloe vera as a treatment for osteoarthritis : a summary." *British Journal of Community Nursing* 15, no. 6 (2010) : 280-2. http://www.ncbi.nlm.nih.gov/pubmed/20679979 (accessed April 18, 2012).

[42] Davis, Robert H., Leitner, Mark G., Russo, Joseph M., & Matro, Nicholas P. (1987). Biological activity of Aloe vera. *Med. Sci. Res, 15*, 235.

[43] Davis, Robert H. (Ph.D.), Shipiro, Eugene, & Agnew, Patrick S. (1985, May). Topical effect of Aloe with ribonucleic acid and vitamin C on adjuvant arthritis. *Journal of the American Podiatry Association,* 75(5), 229-237.

[44] Dahmen U, Gu YL, Dirsch O, et al. Boswellic acid, a potent antiinflammatory drug, inhibits rejection to the same extent as high dose steroids. *Transplant Proc.* Feb-Mar 2001;33(1-2):539-541.

[45] Safayhi H, Boden SE, Schweizer S, et al. Concentration-dependent potentiating and inhibitory effects of Boswellia extracts on 5-lipoxygenase product formation in stimulated PMNL. *Planta Med.* Mar 2000;66(2):110-113.

[46] Safayhi H, Mack T, Sabieraj J, et al. Boswellic acids : novel, specific, nonredox inhibitors of 5-lipoxygenase. *J Pharmacol Exp Ther.* Jun 1992;261(3):1143-1146.

[47] Sengupta K, Alluri KV, Satish AR, et al. A double blind, randomized, placebo controlled study of the efficacy and safety of 5-Loxin(R) for treatment of osteoarthritis of the knee. *Arthritis Res Ther.* Jul 30 2008;10(4):R85.

[48] Zhang WY, Li Wan Po A. The effectiveness of topically applied capsaicin. *Eur J Clin Pharmacol.* 1994;46:517-522.

[49] Deal CL, et al. Treatment of arthritis with topical capsaicin : a double-blind trial. *Clin Ther* 1991;13:383-95.

[50] McCarthy, GM, and DJ McCarty. "Effect of topical capsaicin in the therapy of painful osteoarthritis of the hands." *Journal of Rheumatology* 19, no. 4 (1992) : 604-7.

[51] Hardin SR. Cat's claw : an Amazonian vine decreases inflammation in osteoarthritis. *Complement Ther Clin Pract.* 2007 Feb;13(1):25-8.

[52]   Piscoya J, Rodriguez Z, Bustamante SA, et al. Efficacy and safety of freeze-dried cat's claw in osteoarthritis of the knee : mechanisms of action of the species Uncaria guianensis. *Inflamm.Res* 2001;50(9):442-448.

[53]   Sandoval M, et al. Anti-inflammatory and antioxidant activities of cat's claw (Uncaria tomentosa and Uncaria guianensis) are independent of their alkaloid content. *Phytomedicine* 2002;9:325-37.

[54]   Staiger, C. "Comfrey : A Clinical Overview." *Phytotherapy Research* E pub ahead of print (2012). http://www.ncbi.nlm.nih.gov/pubmed/22359388 (accessed May 1, 2012).

[55]   Grube B, Grunwald J, Krug L, Staiger C. Efficacy of comfrey root (Symphyti offic. radix) extract ointment in the treatment of patients with painful osteoarthritis of the knee : results of a double-blind randomised, bicenter, placebo-controlled trial. *Phytomedicine.* 2007;14(1):2-10.

[56]   Grube, B, et al. "Efficacy of a comfrey root (Symphyti offic. radix) extract ointment in the treatment of patients with painful osteoarthritis of the knee : results of a double-blind, randomised, bicenter, placebo-controlled trial." *Phytomedicine* 14, no. 1 (2007) : 2-10. http://www.ncbi.nlm.nih.gov/pubmed/17169543 (accessed April 17, 2012).

[57]   Giannetti BM, Staiger C, Bulitta M, Predel HG. Efficacy and safety of a Comfrey root extract ointment in the treatment of acute upper or low back pain : results of a double-blind, randomised, placebo-controlled, multi-centre trial. *Br J Sports Med.* 2009;44(9):637-41.

[58]   Gagnier JJ, van Tulder MW, Berman B, et al. Herbal medicine for low back pain. *Spine* 2007;32(1):82-92.

[59]   Wegener T, Lupke NP. Treatment of patients with arthrosis of hip or knee with an aqueous extract of devil's claw (Harpagophytum procumbens DC.). *Phytother Res.* 2003 Dec;17(10):1165-72.

[60]   Warnock, M, et al. "Effectiveness and safety of Devil's Claw tablets in patients with general rheumatic disorders." *Phytotherapy Research* 21, no. 12 (2007) : 1228-33. http://www.ncbi.nlm.nih.gov/pubmed/17886223 (accessed April 24, 2012).

[61] Inaba, K, et al. "Inhibitory effects of devil's claw (secondary root of Harpagophytum procumbens) extract and harpagoside on cytokine production in mouse macrophages." *Journal of Natural Medicines* 64, no. 2 (2010) : 219-22. http://www.ncbi.nlm.nih.gov/pubmed/20177800 (accessed April 25, 2012).

[62] Chantre P, Cappelaere A, Leblan D, et al. Efficacy and tolerance of Harpagophytum procumbens versus diacerhein in treatment of osteoarthritis. *Phytomedicine* 2000;7(3):177-183.

[63] Kim, HA, et al. "Anti-arthritic effect of ginsenoside Rb1 on collagen induced arthritis in mice." *International Immunopharmacology* 7, no. 10 (2007) : 1286-91.

[64] Kim, KR, et al. "Red ginseng saponin extract attenuates murine collagen-induced arthritis by reducing pro-inflammatory responses and matrix metalloproteinase-3 expression." *Biological and pharmaceutical bulletin* 33, no. 4 (2010). http://www.ncbi.nlm.nih.gov/pubmed/20410593 (accessed April 16, 2012).

[65] Lee, Davy CW, et al. "Bioactivity-guided identification and cell signaling technology to delineate the immunomodulatory effects of Panax ginseng on human promonocytic U937 cells." *Journal of Translational Medicine* 7, no. 34 (2009):

[66] Davydov M, Krikorian AD. (October 2000). "Eleutherococcus senticosus (Rupr. & Maxim.) Maxim. (Araliaceae) as an adaptogen : a closer look". *Journal of Ethnopharmacology* 72(3) : 345–393

[67] Randall C, Randall H, Dobbs F, Hutton C, Sanders H. Randomized controlled trial of nettle sting for treatment of base-of-thumb pain. *J R Soc Med.* 2000 Jun;93(6):305-9.

[68] Jacquet A, Girodet PO, Pariente A, et al. Phytalgic(R), a food supplement, vs placebo in patients with osteoarthritis of the knee or hip : a randomised double-blind placebo-controlled clinical trial. *Arthritis Res Ther.* 2009;11(6):R192.

[69] Riehemann, K, et al. "Plant extracts from stinging nettle (Urtica dioica), an antirheumatic remedy, inhibit the proinflammatory transcription factor NF-kappaB." *FEBS Letters* 442, no. 1 (1999) : 89-94. http://www.ncbi.nlm.nih.gov/pubmed/9923611 (accessed May 2, 2012).

[70] Deodhar SD, Sethi R, Srimal RC. Preliminary study on antirheumatic activity of curcumin (diferuloyl methane). *Indian J Med Res.* 1980;71:632-634.

[71] Funk, JL, et al. "Efficacy and mechanism of action of turmeric supplements in the treatment of experimental arthritis." *Arthritis and rheumatism* 54, no. 11 (2006) : 3452-64. http://www.ncbi.nlm.nih.gov/pubmed/17075840 (accessed May 9, 2012).

[72] Kuptniratsaikul V, Thanakhumtorn S, Chinswangwatanakul P, et al. Efficacy and safety of Curcuma domestica extracts in patients with knee osteoarthritis. *J Altern Complement Med.* Aug 2009;15(8):891-897.

[73] Yun JM, Jialal I, Devaraj S. Epigenetic regulation of high glucose-induced proinflammatory cytokine production in monocytes by curcumin. *J Nutr Biochem.* May 2011;22(5):450-458.

[74] Hong J, Bose M, Ju J, et al. Modulation of arachidonic acid metabolism by curcumin and related beta-diketone derivatives : effects on cytosolic phospholipase A(2), cyclooxygenases and 5-lipoxygenase. *Carcinogenesis.* 2004;25(9):1671-1679.

[75] Biegert C, Wagner I, Ludtke R, et al. Efficacy and safety of willow bark extract in the treatment of osteoarthritis and rheumatoid arthritis : results of 2 randomized double-blind controlled trials. *J.Rheumatol.* 2004;31(11):2121-2130.

[76] Chrubasik S, Kunzel O, Model A, et al. Treatment of low back pain with a herbal or synthetic anti-rheumatic : a randomized controlled study. Willow bark extract for low back pain. *Rheumatology* (Oxford) 2001;40(12):1388-1393.

[77] Schmid B, Ludtke R, Selbmann HK, et al. Efficacy and tolerability of a standardized willow bark extract in patients with osteoarthritis : randomized placebo-controlled, double blind clinical trial. *Phytother Res* 2001;15(4):344-350.

[78] Hafstrom I, Ringertz B, Spangberg A, et al. A vegan diet free of gluten improves the signs and symptoms of rheumatoid arthritis : the effects on arthritis correlate with a reduction in antibodies to food antigens. *Rheumatology* (Oxford). 2001;40(10):1175-1179.

79   Campbell, T. Colin, and Thomas M. Campbell. *The China study :
     the most comprehensive study of nutrition ever conducted and the
     startling implications for diet, weight loss and long-term health.*
     Dallas, Tex. : BenBella Books, 2005.

80   McDougall J, Bruce B, Spiller G, Westerdahl J, McDougall M. Effects
     of a very low-fat, vegan diet in subjects with rheumatoid arthritis. *J
     Altern Complement Med.* 2002;8(1):71-75.

81   Hanninen, Kaartinen K, Rauma AL, Nenonen M, Torronen R,
     Hakkinen AS, Adlercreutz H, Laakso J. Antioxidants in vegan diet and
     rheumatic disorders. *Toxicology.* 2000;155(1-3):45-53.

82   About Organic Produce.   http://www.ocf.berkeley.edu/~lhom/
     organictext.html. Accessed 10/5/2012.

83   Welch, Alisa A, et al. "Urine pH is an indicator of dietary acid–base
     load, fruit and vegetables and meat intakes : results from the
     European Prospective Investigation into Cancer and Nutrition
     (EPIC)-Norfolk population study." *British Journal of Nutrition* 99
     (2007) : 1335-1343. http://journals.cambridge.org/action/display
     Abstract?fromPage=online&aid=1850160 (accessed May 15, 2012)

84   Dawson-Hughes, Bess,et al. "Treatment with Potassium Bicarbonate
     Lowers Calcium Excretion and Bone Resorption in Older Men and
     Women." *The Journal of Clinical Endocrinology & Metabolism* 94,
     no. 1 (2009) : 96-102.http://jccm.endojournals.org/content/94/
     1/96.abstract?maxtoshow=&HITS=10&hits=10&RESULTFORMAT
     =1&author1=dawson-hughes&andorexacttitle=and&andorexactti
     tleabs=and&andorexactfulltext=and&searchid=1&FIRSTINDEX=0
     &sortspec=relevance&fdate=1/1/2009&tdate=5/31/20 (accessed
     May 14, 2012).

85   Kawaguchi, K, et al. . "Effects of antioxidant polyphenols on
     TNF-alpha-related diseases." *Current Topics in Medicinal Chemistry*
     11, no. 14 (2011) : 1767-79. http://www.ncbi.nlm.nih.gov/
     pubmed/21506932 (accessed May 15, 2012).

86   Pattison, Dorothy J, et al. "Dietary ß-cryptoxanthin and inflammatory
     polyarthritis : results from a population-based prospective study."
     The American Journal of Clinical Nutrition 82, no. 2 (2005) : 451-455,.
     pubmed.gov (accessed May 14, 2012).

87   Wang Y, et al. "The effect of nutritional supplements on osteoarthritis."
     Alternative Medical Review 2004, 9:275-296

[88] Lahiri, M, et al. "Modifiable risk factors for RA : prevention, better than cure?." *Rheumatology* 51, no. 3 (2012) : 499-512. http://www.ncbi.nlm.nih.gov/pubmed/22120459 (accessed May 7, 2012).

[89] Seki, T, et al. "Association of serum carotenoids, retinol, and tocopherols with radiographic knee osteoarthritis : possible risk factors in rural Japanese inhabitants." *Journal of Orthopaedic Science* 15, no. 4 (2011) : 477-84. http://www.ncbi.nlm.nih.gov/pubmed/20721715 (accessed May 15, 2012).

[90] Wang, Y,et al. "Effect of antioxidants on knee cartilage and bone in healthy, middle-aged subjects : a cross-sectional study." *Arthritis Research and Therapy* 9, no. R66 (2007). http://arthritis-research.com/content/9/4/R66/ (accessed May 14, 2012).

[91] Brambila-Tapia, AJ, et al. "MTHFR C677T, MTHFR A1298C, and OPG A163G polymorphisms in Mexican patients with rheumatoid arthritis and osteoporosis." *Disease Markers* 32, no. 2 (2012) : 109-14.

[92] Gough, KR, et al. "Folic-acid Deficiency in Rheumatoid Arthritis." *British Medical Journal* 1, no. 5377 (1964) : 212–217.

[93] Das A, Jr., Hammad TA. Efficacy of a combination of FCHG49 glucosamine hydrochloride, TRH122 low molecular weight sodium chondroitin sulfate and manganese ascorbate in the management of knee osteoarthritis. *Osteoarthritis Cartilage.* 2000;8(5):343-350.

[94] Leffler CT, Philippi AF, Leffler SG, Mosure JC, Kim PD. Glucosamine, chondroitin, and manganese ascorbate for degenerative joint disease of the knee or low back : a randomized, double-blind, placebo-controlled pilot study. *Mil Med.* 1999;164(2):85-91

[95] Hill J, Bird HA, Fenn GC, Lee CE, Woodward M, Wright V. A double-blind crossover study to compare lysine acetyl salicylate (Aspergesic) with ibuprofen in the treatment of rheumatoid arthritis. *J Clin Pharm Ther.* 1990;15(3):205-211.

[96] Jensen, GS,et al. "In vitro and in vivo antioxidant and anti-inflammatory capacities of an antioxidant-rich fruit and berry juice blend. Results of a pilot and randomized, double-blinded, placebo-controlled, crossover study." *Journal of Agricultural and Food Chemistry* 56, no. 18 (2008): : 8326-33. http://www.ncbi.nlm.nih.gov/pubmed?term=In%20Vitro%20and%20in%20Vivo%20Antioxidant%20and%20Anti-Inflammatory%20Capacities%20of%20an%20Antioxidant-Rich%20Fruit%20and%20Berry%20Juice%20Blend (accessed April 9, 2012).

97   "Schauss , AG, et al. "Antioxidant Capacity and Other Bioactivities of the Freeze-Dried Amazonian Palm Berry." *Journal of Agricultural and Food Chemistry;*" 54, no. 22 (2006) : :8604-10.

98   Jensen, GS, et al. "Pain reduction and improvement in range of motion after daily consumption of an açai (Euterpe oleracea Mart.) pulp-fortified polyphenolic-rich fruit and berry juice blend." *Journal of Medicinal Food* 14, no. 7-8 (2011): 702-11.

99   Hassimotto NM, Genovese MI, Lajolo FM, et al. Antioxidant activity of dietary fruits, vegetables, and commercial frozen fruit pulps. *J Agric Food Chem.* 2005;53:2928–35.

100   Pattison, D, et al. "Vitamin C and the risk of developing inflammatory polyarthritis: prospective nested case-control study." *Annals of Rheumatic Disease* 36, no. 7 (2004) : 277-91.

101   Hanamura T, Hagiwara T, Kawagishi H. Structural and functional characterization of polyphenols isolated from acerola (Malpighia emarginata DC.) fruit. *Biosci. Biotechnol. Biochem.* 2005;69(2):280-286.

102   "Aronia melanocarpa phenolics and their antioxidant activity", Jan Oszmianski and Aneta Wojdylo, *European Food Research and Technology,* Volume 221, Number 6, 809-813.

103   Zapolska-Downar, D, et al. "Aronia melanocarpa fruit extract exhibits anti-inflammatory activity in human aortic endothelial cells." *European Journal of Nutrition* e-pub ahead of print (2011). http://www.ncbi.nlm.nih.gov/pubmed/21863241 (accessed April 8, 2012).

104   Qin, B, and RA Anderson. "An extract of chokeberry attenuates weight gain and modulates insulin, adipogenic and inflammatory signalling pathways in epididymal adipose tissue of rats fed a fructose-rich diet." *British Journal of Nutrition* 6 (2011) : 1-7.

105   Zadok D, et al. The effect of anthocyanosides on night vision tests. *Invest Ophthalmol Vis Sci* 1997;38(suppl):633.

106   Lietti A, et al. Studies on Vaccinium myrtillus anthocyanosides. I. Vasoprotective and antiinflammatory activity. *Arzneimittelforschung.* 1976;26(5):829-32.

[107] Monboisse JC, Braquet P, Randoux A, et al. Non-enzymatic degradation of acid-soluble calf skin collagen by superoxide ion : Protective effect of flavonoids. *Biochem Pharmacol.* 1983;32:53-58.

[108] Gabor M. Pharmacologic effects of flavonoids on blood vessels. *Angiologica.* 1972;9:355-374.

[109] Wu, Dayong, et al. "Effect of dietary supplementation with black currant seed oil on the immune response of healthy elderly subjects." *American Journal of Clinical Nutrition* 70 (1999) : 536–43. http://www.ajcn.org/content/70/4/536.full.pdf (accessed April 8, 2012).

[110] Bishayee, A, et al. "Black currant phytoconstituents exert chemoprevention of diethylnitrosamine-initiated hepatocarcinogenesis by suppression of the inflammatory response." *Molecular carcinogenesis* 10.1002/mc.21860 (2011): .

[111] Lyall, KA, et al. "Short-term blackcurrant extract consumption modulates exercise-induced oxidative stress and lipopolysaccharide-stimulated inflammatory responses." *American Journal of Physiology - Regulatory, Integrative and Comparative Physiology* 297, no. 1 (2009): :R70-81.

[112] Netzel M, Strass G, Janssen M, et al. Bioactive anthocyanins detected in human urine after ingestion of blackcurrant juice. *J Environ.Pathol Toxicol Oncol* 2001;20(2):89-95.

[113] Netzel M, Strass G, Janssen M, et al. Bioactive anthocyanins detected in human urine after ingestion of blackcurrant juice. *J Environ. Pathol Toxicol Oncol* 2001;20(2):89-95.

[114] Blomhoff R. [Antioxidants and oxidative stress]. Tidsskr. *Nor Laegeforen.* 6-17-2004;124(12):1643-1645.

[115] Pergola, C, et al. "Inhibition of nitricoxidebiosynthesis by anthocyaninfraction of blackberryextract." *Nitric Oxide-Biology and Chemistry* 15, no. 1 (2006) : 30-39. http://www.sciencedirect.com/science/article/pii/S1089860305001515 (accessed April 16, 2012).

[116] Halvorsen, Bente L. et al, . "Content of redox-active compounds (ie, antioxidants) in foods consumed in the United States." *The American Journal of Medical Nutrition* 84, no. 1 (2006) : 95-135. http://www.ajcn.org/content/84/1/95.full?sid=a885ee97-3604-4a7b-b8d7-6222ece600fb (accessed April 9, 2012).

[117] Neto, CC. "Cranberry and blueberry : evidence for protective effects against cancer and vascular diseases." *Molecular Nutrition & Food Research* 51, no. 6 (2007) : 652-64.

[118] DeFuria J, Bennett G, Strissel KJ et al. Dietary . Dietary Blueberry Attenuates Whole-Body Insulin Resistance in High Fat-Fed Mice by Reducing Adipocyte Death and Its Inflammatory Sequelae. *J Nutr.* 2009 August; 139(8) : 1510-1516. doi : 10.3945/jn.109.105155. 2009.

[119] Hurst RD, Wells RW, Hurst SM et al. Blueberry fruit polyphenolics suppress oxidative stress-induced skeletal muscle cell damage in vitro. *Mol Nutr Food Res.* 2010 Mar;54(3):353-63. 2010.

[120] Keyvan Dastmalchi, Gema Flores, Vanya Petrova, Paola Pedraza-Peñalosa, Edward J. Kennelly. Edible Neotropical Blueberries : Antioxidant and Compositional Fingerprint Analysis. *Journal of Agricultural and Food Chemistry,* 2011; 59 (7) : 3020

[121] Jin-Ran Chen, Oxana P Lazarenko, Xianli Wu, Jie Kang, Michael L Blackburn, Kartik Shankar, Thomas M Badger, Martin JJ Ronis. Dietary-induced serum phenolic acids promote bone growth via p38 MAPK/β-catenin canonical Wnt signaling. *Journal of Bone and Mineral Research,* 2010; 25 (11) : 2399

[122] Justi KC, Visentainer JV, Evelázio de Souza N, Matsushita M. "Nutritional composition and vitamin C stability in stored camu-camu (Myrciaria dubia) pulp." *Arch Latinoam Nutr.* 2000 Dec;50(4):405-8.

[123] Yazawa K, Suga K, Honma A, Shirosaki M, Koyama T. Anti-Inflammatory Effects of Seeds of the Tropical Fruit Camu-Camu (Myrciaria dubia). *J Nutr Sci Vitaminol* (Tokyo). 2011;57(1):104-7.

[124] Inoue , T, et al. "Tropical fruit camu-camu (Myrciaria dubia) has anti-oxidative and anti-inflammatory properties." *Journal of Cardiology* 52, no. 2 (2008) : 127-32. http://www.ncbi.nlm.nih.gov/pubmed?term=%22camu%20camu%22%20inflammation (accessed April 9, 2012)

[125] Jacob, Robert A, et al. "Consumption of Cherries Lowers Plasma Urate in Healthy Women." *The Journal of Nutrition* 133, no. 6 (2003) : 1826-1829.

[126] Kelley, Darshan. "Consumption of Bing Sweet Cherries Lowers Circulating Concentrations of Inflammation Markers in Healthy Men and Women." *The Journal of Nutrition* 136, no. 4 (2006) : 981-986.

[127] "CanCherriesRelieveThePainOfOsteoarthritis?."*ScienceDaily.*http://
www.sciencedaily.com/releases/2009/03/090319164327.htm
(accessed April 13, 2012).

[128] Beverly K, Basu A and Lucas EA. Anti-inflammatory effects of cranberry
juice in lipopolysaccharide (LPS)-stimulated RAW 264.7 murine
macrophage cells. *FASEB J.* 2008 22:890.8 [Meeting Abstract] 2008.

[129] Pappas E and Schaich KM. Phytochemicals of cranberries and
cranberry products : characterization, potential health effects, and
processing stability. *Crit Rev Food Sci Nutr.*

[130] Viskelis, P, et al. "Anthocyanins, antioxidative, and antimicrobial
properties of American cranberry (Vaccinium macrocarpon Ait.)
and their press cakes." *Journal of Food Science* 74, no. 2 (2009) :
C157-61.

[131] Ruel G, Pomerleau S, Couture P, Lemieux S, Lamarche B, Couillard
C. Low-calorie cranberry juice supplementation reduces plasma
oxidized LDL and cell adhesion molecule concentrations in men.
Brit J Nutr. 2008;99(2):352-9.

[132] J Alt Compl Mod 1995 : 1:361-69 2. Youdim KA, Martin A, Joseph JA.
Incorporation of the elderberry anthocyanins by endothelial cells
increases protection against oxidative stress. *Free Radical Biol Med*
2000 : 29:51 60

[133] Zafra-Stone, S,et al. "Berry anthocyanins as novel antioxidants in
human health and disease prevention." *Molecular Nutrition & Food
Research* 51, no. 6 (2007) : 675-83.

[134] Charlebois, D. "Elderberry as a Medicinal Plant." http://www.
hort.purdue.edu.   www.hort.purdue.edu/newcrop/ncnu07/pdfs/
charlebois284-292.pdf (accessed April 9, 2012).

[135] Reifen, R, et al. "Lycopene supplementation attenuates the
inflammatory status of colitis in a rat model." *International Journal for
Vitamin and Nutrition Research* 71, no. 6 (2001) : 347-51. http://www.
ncbi.nlm.nih.gov/pubmed/11840838 (accessed April 12, 2012).

[136] Riccioni, G, et al. "Novel phytonutrient contributors to antioxidant
protection against cardiovascular disease." *Nutrition.* (2012) : .
http://www.ncbi.nlm.nih.gov/pubmed/22480801 (accessed April
13, 2012).

[137] Wu, SJ, et al. "Antioxidant activities of some common ingredients of traditional chinese medicine, Angelica sinensis, Lycium barbarum and Poria cocos." *Phtotherapy Research* 18, no. 12 (2004) : 1008-12.

[138] Amagase , H, et al. "Lycium barbarum (goji) juice improves in vivo antioxidant biomarkers in serum of healthy adults." Nutrition Research29, no. 1 (2009) : 19-25.

[139] Zhang, Z,et al. "Comparative evaluation of the antioxidant effects of the natural vitamin C analog 2-O-β-D-glucopyranosyl-L-ascorbic acid isolated from Goji berry fruit." *Archives of Pharmacal Research* 34, no. 5 (2011) : 801-10.

[140] Amagase H, Nance DM. A randomized, double-blind, placebo-controlled, clinical study of the general effects of a standardized Lycium barbarum (Goji) Juice, GoChi. *J Altern Complement Med.* 2008 May;14(4):403-12.

[141] Gan L, Zhang SH, Liu Q, Xu HB. A polysaccharide-protein complex from Lycium barbarum upregulates cytokine expression in human peripheral blood mononuclear cells. *Eur J Pharmacol.* 2003;471:217-22.

[142] Ko, SH, et al. "Comparison of the antioxidant activities of nine different fruits in human plasma." *Journal of Medicinal Food* 8, no. 1 (2005) : 41-6.

[143] Iwasawa, H, et al. "Anti-oxidant effects of kiwi fruit in vitro and in vivo." *Biological and Pharmaceutical Bulletin* 34, no. 1 (2011) : 128-34. http://www.ncbi.nlm.nih.gov/pubmed/21212530 (accessed April 15, 2012).

[144] Collins BH, Horska A, Hotten PM, et al. Kiwifruit protects against oxidative DNA damage in human cells and in vitro. *Nutr Cancer* 2001;39(1):148-53 2001. PMID:13330.

[145] Dawczynski, C, et al. "Incorporation of n-3 PUFA and γ-linolenic acid in blood lipids and red blood cell lipids together with their influence on disease activity in patients with chronic inflammatory arthritis -- a randomized controlled human intervention trial." *Lipids in Health and Diseases* 10, no. 130 (2011) : .

[146] Garrido-Suárez, BB, et al. "A Mangifera indica L. extract could be used to treat neuropathic pain and implication of mangiferin." *Molecules* 15, no. 12 (2010) : 9035-45.

147   Garrido, G, et al. "In vivo and in vitro anti-inflammatory activity of Mangifera indica L. extract (VIMANG)." *Pharmacological Research* 50, no. 2 (2004) : 143-9. http://www.ncbi.nlm.nih.gov/pubmed/15177302 (accessed April 17, 2012).

148   Kumar, IV, et al. "Swertia chirayita mediated modulation of interleukin-1beta, interleukin-6, interleukin-10, interferon-gamma, and tumor necrosis factor-alpha in arthritic mice." *Immunopharmacology and Immunotoxicology* 25, no. 4 (2012) : 573-83. http://www.ncbi.nlm.nih.gov/pubmed/14686799 (accessed April 22, 2012).

149   Cui, J, et al. "New medicinal properties of mangostins : analgesic activity and pharmacological characterization of active ingredients from the fruit hull of Garcinia mangostana L." *Pharmacology, Biochemistry and Behavior* 95, no. 2 (2010) : 166-72. http://www.ncbi.nlm.nih.gov/pubmed/20064550 (accessed April 17, 2012).

150   Chen, LG, et al. "Anti-inflammatory activity of mangostins from Garcinia mangostana." *Food and Chemical Toxicology* 46, no. 2 (2008) : 688-93. http://www.ncbi.nlm.nih.gov/pubmed/18029076 (accessed April 10, 2012).

151   Nakatani K, et al. Inhibition of cyclooxygenase and prostaglandin E2 synthesis by gamma-mangostin, a xanthone derivative in mangosteen, in C6 rat glioma cells. *Biochem Pharmacol* 2002; 63(1):73-79.

152   Suksamrarn S, et al. Xanthones from the green fruit hulls of Garcinia mangostana. *J Nat Prod* 2002; 65(5):761-763.

153   "NWFP Digest-L." FAO : *Food and Agriculture Organization of the United Nations.* http://www.fao.org/forestry/61458/en/ (accessed April 19, 2012).

154   Ruiz, A, et al. "Polyphenols and antioxidant activity of calafate (Berberis microphylla) fruits and other native berries from Southern Chile." *Journal of Agricultural and Food Chemistry* 58, no. 10 (2010) : 6081-9.

155   Seong, AR, et al. "Delphinidin, a specific inhibitor of histone acetyltransferase, suppresses inflammatory signaling via prevention of NF-κB acetylation in fibroblast-like synoviocyte MH7A cells." *Biochemical and Biophysical Research* 410, no. 3 (2011):581-6. http://www.ncbi.nlm.nih.gov/pubmed?term=Delphinidin%20arthritis (accessed April 17, 2012).

[156] Hidalgo, M. "Potential anti-inflammatory, anti-adhesive, anti/estrogenic, and angiotensin-converting enzyme inhibitory activities of anthocyanins and their gut metabolites." *Genes & Nutrition* 7, no. 2 (2012) : 295-306. http://www.ncbi.nlm.nih.gov/pubmed/22218934 (accessed April 16, 2012).

[157] Wang, Mian-Ying,et al. "Morinda citrifolia L. (noni) improves the Quality of Life in adults with Osteoarthritis."*Functional Foods in Health and Disease* 2 (2011) : 75-90

[158] Kamiya K, et al. Chemical constituents of Morinda citrifolia fruits inhibit copper-induced low-density lipoprotein oxidation. *J Agric Food Chem* 2004; 52(19) : 5843-8.

[159] Su BN, et al. Chemical constituents of the fruits of Morinda citrifolia (Noni) and their antioxidant activity. *J Nat Prod* 2005 68(4):592-5.

[160] Sang S, et al. Flavonol glycosides and novel iridoid glycoside from the leaves of Morinda citrifolia. *J Agric Food Chem* 2001 49(9):4478-81.

[161] Basar, Simia, et al. "Analgesic and antiinflammatory activity of Morinda citrifolia L. (Noni) fruit." Phytotherapy Research 24, no. 1 (2010) : 38-42.

[162] Adams LS, Seeram NP, Aggarwal BB, Takada Y, Sand D, Heber D. Pomegranate juice, total pomegranate ellagitannins, and punicalagin suppress inflammatory cell signaling in colon cancer cells. *J Agric Food Chem.* Feb 8 2006;54(3):980-985.

[163] Aviram M, Dornfeld L, Rosenblat M, et al. Pomegranate juice consumption reduces oxidative stress, atherogenic modifications to LDL, and platelet aggregation : studies in humans and in atherosclerotic apolipoprotein E-deficient mice. *Am J Clin Nutr* 2000;71(5):1062-1076.

[164] Balbir-Gurman , A, et al. "Consumption of pomegranate decreases serum oxidative stress and reduces disease activity in patients with active rheumatoid arthritis : a pilot study." *The Israel Medical Association Journal* 13, no. 8 (2011) : 474-9. http://www.ncbi.nlm. nih.gov/pubmed/21910371 (accessed April 16, 2012).

[165] Rasheed, Z, et al. "Pomegranate extract inhibits the interleukin-1β-induced activation of MKK-3, p38α-MAPK and transcription factor RUNX-2 in human osteoarthritis chondrocytes." *Arthritis Research and Therapy* 12, no. 5 (2010) : R195.

[166] Cerhan, James R, et al. "Antioxidant Micronutrients and Risk of Rheumatoid Arthritis in a Cohort of Older Women." *American Journal of Epidemiology* 157, no. 4 (2003) : 345-354. http://aje.oxfordjournals. org/content/157/4/345.full (accessed April 17, 2012).

[167] Chen, G, et al. "Effect and mechanism of total flavonoids of orange peel on rat adjuvant arthritis." *Zhongguo Zhong Yao Za Zhi.* 35, no. 10 (2010) : 1298-301. http://www.ncbi.nlm.nih.gov/pubmed/20707201 (accessed April 17, 2012).

[168] Galati EM, Monforte MT, Kirjavainen S, et al. Biological effects of hesperidin, a citrus flavonoid. (Note I) : antiinflammatory and analgesic activity. *Farmaco* 1994

[169] Pattison, D, et al. "Vitamin C and the risk of developing inflammatory polyarthritis : prospective nested case-control study." *Annals of Rheumatic Disease* 36, no. 7 (2004) : 277-91.

[170] Agarwal S, Rao AV. Carotenoids and chronic diseases. *Drug Metabol Drug Interact* 2000;17(1-4):189-210 2000. PMID:15130.

[171] Marotta, F, et al. "Nutraceutical strategy in aging : targeting heat shock protein and inflammatory profile through understanding interleukin-6 polymorphism." *Annals of the New York Academy of Sciences* 1119 (2007) : 196-202.

[172] Montanher , AB, et al. "Effect of Passiflora edulis (passion fruit) extract on rats' bladder wound healing : morphological study." *Journal of Ethnopharmacology* 109, no. 2 (2007) : 281-8.

[173] Farid , R, et al. "Oral intake of purple passion fruit peel extract reduces pain and stiffness and improves physical function in adult patients with knee osteoarthritis." *Nutrition Research* 30, no. 9 (2010) : 601-6. http://www.ncbi.nlm.nih.gov/pubmed?term=passion%20 fruit%20arthritis (accessed April 16, 2012).

[174] Piotrowska, H, M Kucinska, and M Murias. "Biological activity of piceatannol : Leaving the shadow of resveratrol." *Mutation Research* E pub ahead of Print (2011) :

[175] Onken JE, Greer PK, Calingaert B, et al. Bromelain treatment decreases secretion of pro-inflammatory cytokines and chemokines by colon biopsies in vitro. *Clin Immunol.* Mar 2008;126(3):345-352.

[176] Secor ER, Carson WF, Singh A, et al. Oral Bromelain Attenuates Inflammation in an Ovalbumin-induced Murine Model of Asthma. *Evid Based Complement Alternat Med.* Mar 2008;5(1):61-69.

[177] Walker AF, et al. Bromelain reduces mild acute knee pain and improves well-being in a dose-dependent fashion in an open study of otherwise healthy adults. *Phytomedicine* 2002 Dec;9(8):681-6.

[178] Klein, G, et al. "Inhibitory effect of enzyme therapy and combination therapy with cyclosporin A on collagen-induced arthritis." *Clinical and Experimental Rheumatology* 24, no. 1 (2006) : 25-30. http://www.ncbi.nlm.nih.gov/pubmed/16539815 (accessed April 2, 2012).

[179] Desser, L, et al. "Oral therapy with proteolytic enzymes decreases excessive TGF-beta levels in human blood." *Cancer Chemotherapy and Pharmacology* 47 (2001) : S10-15.

[180] Nakatani N, Kayano S, Kikuzaki H, et al. Identification, quantitative determination, and antioxidative activities of chlorogenic acid isomers in prune (Prunus domestica L.). *J Agric Food Chem* 2000 Nov;48(11):5512-6 2000. PMID:13580.

[181] Stacewicz-Sapuntzakis M, Bowen PE, Hussain EA, et al. Chemical composition and potential health effects of prunes : a functional food. *Crit Rev Food Sci Nutr* 2001 May;41(4):251-86 2001. PMID:13590.

[182] Guedes, AC, et al. "Microalgae as sources of carotenoids." *Marine Drugs* 9, no. 4 (2011) : 625-44.

[183] Zhou, X, et al. "Cutting edge : all-trans retinoic acid sustains the stability and function of natural regulatory T cells in an inflammatory milieu." *Journal of Immunology* 185, no. 5 (2010) : 2675-9.

[184] Kijlstra , A, et al. "Lutein : More than just a filter for blue light." *Progress In Retinal And Eye Research* March 21 (2012). http://www.ncbi.nlm.nih.gov/pubmed/22465791 (accessed April 9, 2012).

[185] Fahim, AT, et al. "Effect of pumpkin-seed oil on the level of free radical scavengers induced during adjuvant-arthritis in rats." *Pharmacological Research* 31, no. 1 (1995) : 73-9

[186] Atta UR, et al. New antioxidant and antimicrobial ellagic acid derivatives from Pteleopsis hylodendron. *Planta Medica* 2001;67:335-9.

[187] Festa F, et al. Strong antioxidant activity of ellagic acid in mammalian cells in vitro revealed by the comet assay. *Anticancer Research* 2001;21:3903-8.

[188] Rogerio, Alexandre P, et al. "Anti-inflammatory, analgesic and anti-oedematous effects of Lafoensia pacari extract and ellagic acid." *Journal of Pharmacy and Pharmacology* 58, no. 9 (2006) : 1265–1273.

[189] Jean-Gilles, D. "Anti-inflammatory Effects of Polyphenolic-Enriched Red Raspberry Extract in an Antigen-Induced Arthritis Rat Model." *Journal of Agricultural Food and Chemistry* E-published ahead of print (2011) :. http://www.ncbi.nlm.nih.gov/pubmed?term=raspberry%20 arthritis (accessed April 8, 2012).

[190] Basu A, Fu DX, Wilkinson M et al. Strawberries decrease atherosclerotic markers in subjects with metabolic syndrome. *Nutr Res.* 2010 Jul;30(7): 462-9. 2010.

[191] Ellis, CL, et al. "Attenuation of meal-induced inflammatory and thrombotic responses in overweight men and women after 6-week daily strawberry (Fragaria) intake. A randomized placebo-controlled trial." *Journal of Atherosclerosis and Thrombosis* 18, no. 4 (2011) : 318-27.

[192] Burton-Freeman B, Linares A, Hyson D et al. . Strawberry Modulates LDL Oxidation and Postprandial Lipemia in Response to High-Fat Meal in Overweight Hyperlipidemic Men and Women. *J. Am. Coll. Nutr.,* Feb 2010; 29 : 46 - 54. 2010.

[193] Kanodia L, Borgohain M, and Das S. Effect of fruit extract of Fragaria vesca L. on experimentally induced inflammatory bowel disease in albino rats. *Indian J Pharmacol.* 2011 Feb;43(1):18-21. 2011.

[194] Edwards AJ, Vinyard BT, Wiley ER et al. Consumption of watermelon juice increases plasma concentrations of lycopene and beta-carotene in humans. *J Nutr* 2003 Apr;133(4):1043-50 2003.

[195] Reifen, R, et al. "Lycopene supplementation attenuates the inflammatory status of colitis in a rat model." *International Journal for Vitamin and Nutrition Research* 71, no. 6 (2001) : 347-51. http://www. ncbi.nlm.nih.gov/pubmed/11840838 (accessed April 12, 2012).

[196] De Pablo, P, et al. "Antioxidants and other novel cardiovascular risk factors in subjects with rheumatoid arthritis in a large population sample." *Arthritis and Rheumatism* 57, no. 6 (2007) : 953-62.

[197] Choi, WJ, et al. "Independent association of serum retinol and β-carotene levels with hyperuricemia : A national population study." *Arthritis Care & Research* 64, no. 3 (2012) : 389-96. http://www. ncbi.nlm.nih.gov/pubmed?term=Independent%20association%20 of%20serum%20retinol%20and%20%CE%B2-carotene%20 levels%20with%20hyperuricemia%3A%20A%20national%20 population%20study (accessed April 22, 2012).

[198] Hong, YH, et al. "Ethyl acetate extracts of alfalfa (Medicago sativa L.) sprouts inhibit lipopolysaccharide-induced inflammation in vitro and in vivo." *Journal of Biomedical Science* 16, no. 64 (2009). http://www. ncbi.nlm.nih.gov/pubmed/19594948 (accessed April 10, 2012).

[199] Kole, L, et al. "Biochanin-A, an isoflavon, showed anti-proliferative and anti-inflammatory activities through the inhibition of iNOS expression, p38-MAPK and ATF-2 phosphorylation and blocking NFκB nuclear translocation." *European Journal of Pharmacology* 653, no. 1-3 (2011) : 8-15.

[200] Neogi T, Booth SL, Zhang YQ, et al. Low vitamin K status is associated with osteoarthritis in the hand and knee. *Arthritis Rheum* 2006;54:1255–61.

[201] Oka, H. "Association of low dietary vitamin K intake with radiographic knee osteoarthritis in the Japanese elderly population : dietary survey in a population-based cohort of the ROAD study." *Journal of Orthopaedic Science* 14, no. 6 (2009) : 687-92. http://www.ncbi. nlm.nih.gov/pubmed/19997813 (accessed April 10, 2012).

[202] Lee do, Y, et al. "Anti-inflammatory effects of Asparagus cochinchinensis extract in acute and chronic cutaneous inflammation." *Journal of Ethnopharmacology* 121, no. 1 (2009) : 28-34. http://www.ncbi. nlm.nih.gov/pubmed/18691647 (accessed April 10, 2012).

[203] Sidiq T, Khajuria A, Suden P et al. A novel sarsasapogenin glycoside from Asparagus racemosus elicits protective immune responses against HBsAg. *Immunol Lett.* 2011 Mar 30;135(1-2):129-35. Epub 2010 Oct 28. 2011.

[204] Nwafor , PA, and FK Okwuasaba . "Anti-nociceptive and anti-inflammatory effects of methanolic extract of Asparagus pubescens root in rodents." *Journal of Ethnopharmacology* 84, no. 2-3 (2003) : 125-9.http://www.ncbi.nlm.nih.gov/pubmed?term=asparagus%20 saponin%20inflammation (accessed April 3, 2012)

[205] Yu YM, Wu CH, Tseng CE, Tsai CE, Chang WC. Antioxidative and hypolipidemic effects of barley leaf essence in a rabbit model of atherosclerosis. *Jpn J Pharmacol.* 2002;89:142-148.

[206] 9. Cremer L, Herold A, Avram D, Szegli G. A purified green barley extract with modulatory properties upon TNF alpha and ROS released by human specialized cells isolated from RA patients. *Roum Arch Microbiol Immunol.* 1998;57:231-242.

[207] Subramoniam, A, et al. "Chlorophyll Revisited : Anti-inflammatory Activities of Chlorophyll a and Inhibition of Expression of TNF-α Gene by the Same." *Inflammation* E-pub ahead of print (2011). http://www.ncbi.nlm.nih.gov/pubmed/22038065 (accessed April 9, 2012).

[208] Kong, JS, et al. "Inhibition of synovial hyperplasia, rheumatoid T cell activation, and experimental arthritis in mice by sulforaphane, a naturally occurring isothiocyanate." *Arthritis and Rheumatism* 62, no. 1 (2010) : 159-170. http://www.ncbi.nlm.nih.gov/pubmed/20039434 (accessed April 10, 2012).

[209] "Eating broccoli could guard against arthritis." *EurekAlert.* http://www.eurekalert.org/pub_releases/2010-09/uoea-ebc091510.php (accessed April 17, 2012).

[210] Christensen, LP. "Galactolipids as potential health promoting compounds in vegetable foods." *Recent Patents on Food, Nutrition & Agriculture* 1, no. 1 (2009) : 50-8. http://www.ncbi.nlm.nih.gov/pubmed/20653526 (accessed April 9, 2012).

[211] Dey et al. "Dietary phenethylisothiocyanate attenuates bowel inflammation in mice." *BMC Chemical Biology,* 2010; 10 (1) : 4

[212] Lee, YM, et al. "Phenethylisothiocyanate inhibits 12-O-tetradecanoylphorbol-13-acetate-induced inflammatory responses in mouse skin." *Journal of Medicinal Food* 14, no. 4 (2011) : 377-85.

[213] Lee, HJ, YK Park, and MH Kang. "The effect of carrot juice, β-carotene supplementation on lymphocyte DNA damage, erythrocyte antioxidant enzymes and plasma lipid profiles in Korean smoker." *Nutrition Research and Practice* 5, no. 8 (2011) : 540-7. http://www.ncbi.nlm.nih.gov/pubmed/22259679 (accessed April 9, 2012).

[214] Rastmanesh, Reza, et al. "A Pilot Study of Potassium Supplementation in the Treatment of Hypokalemic Patients With Rheumatoid Arthritis : A Randomized, Double-Blinded, Placebo-Controlled Trial." *The Journal of Pain* 9, no. 8 (2008) : 722-731. http://www.jpain.org/article/S1526-5900(08)00497-5/abstract (accessed April 8, 2012).

[215] Agarwal S, Rao AV. Carotenoids and chronic diseases. *Drug Metabol Drug Interact* 2000;17(1-4):189-210 2000. PMID:15130.

[216] Guerrero-Beltrán, CE, et al. "Protective effect of sulforaphane against oxidative stress : Recent advances." *Experimental and Toxicologic Pathology* E-pub ahead of print (2010). http://www.ncbi.nlm.nih.gov/pubmed/21129940 (accessed April 17, 2012).

217   Potapovich, AI, et al. "Plant polyphenols differentially modulate inflammatory responses of human keratinocytes by interfering with activation of transcription factors NFκB and AhR and EGFR-ERK pathway." *Toxicology and Applied Pharmacology* 255, no. 2 (2011) : 138-49. http://www.ncbi.nlm.nih.gov/pubmed/21756928 (accessed April 10, 2012).

218   Dong, L, et al. "Diindolylmethane attenuates experimental arthritis and osteoclastogenesis." *Biochemical Pharmacology* 79, no. 5 (2010) : 715-21. http://www.ncbi.nlm.nih.gov/pubmed?term=3%2C3'-Diindolylmethane%20attenuates%20experimental%20 arthritis%20and%20osteoclastogenesis. (accessed April 3, 2012).

219   Atta AH, Alkofahi A. Anti-nociceptive and anti-inflammatory effects of some Jordanian medicinal plant extracts. *J Ethnopharmacol.* 1998;60:117-124.

220   Dong, L, et al. "Diindolylmethane attenuates experimental arthritis and osteoclastogenesis." *Biochemical Pharmacology* 79, no. 5 (2010) : 715-21. http://www.ncbi.nlm.nih.gov/pubmed?term=3%2C3'-Diindolylmethane%20attenuates%20experimental%20 arthritis%20and%20osteoclastogenesis. (accessed April 3, 2012).

221   Tarozzi A, Morroni F, Merlicco A, et al. Sulforaphane as an inducer of glutathione prevents oxidative stress-induced cell death in a dopaminergic-like neuroblastoma cell line. *J Neurochem.* 2009 Dec;111(5):1161-71. 2009.

222   McAlindon" T.E., et al. "Do antioxidant micronutrients protect against the development and progression of knee arthritis?," *Arthritis and Rheumatism* 39(4):648-656. 1996.

223   Tanira MOM, Shah AH, Mohsin A, et al. Pharmacological and toxicological investigations on Foeniculum vulgare dried fruit extract in experimental animals. *Phytother Res.* 1996;10:33–6.

224   Aggarwa, BB, and S Shishodia. "Suppression of the nuclear factor-kappaB activation pathway by spice-derived phytochemicals: reasoning for seasoning." *Annals of the New York Academy of Sciences* 1030 (2004) : 434-41. http://www.ncbi.nlm.nih.gov/pubmed/15659827 (accessed April 16, 2012).

225   Chainy GB, Manna SK, Chaturvedi MM, Aggarwal BB. Anethole blocks both early and late cellular responses transduced by tumor necrosis factor : effect on NF-kappaB, AP-1, JNK, MAPKK and apoptosis. *Oncogene* 2000 Jun 8;19(25):2943-50 2000. PMID:12930.

[226] Pellegrini N, Chiavaro E, Gardana C et al. Effect of Different Cooking Methods on Color, Phytochemical Concentration, and Antioxidant Capacity of Raw and Frozen Brassica Vegetables. *J. Agric. Food Chem.,* 2010, 58 (7), pp 4310-4321. 2010.

[227] Prawan A, Saw CL, Khor TO et al. Anti-NF-kappaB and anti-inflammatory activities of synthetic isothiocyanates : effect of chemical structures and cellular signaling. *Chem Biol Interact.* 2009 May 15;179(2-3):202-11. 2009.

[228] Tarozzi A, Morroni F, Merlicco A, et al. Sulforaphane as an inducer of glutathione prevents oxidative stress-induced cell death in a dopaminergic-like neuroblastoma cell line. *J Neurochem.* 2009 Dec;111(5):1161-71. 2009.

[229] Zhu H, Jia Z, Zhou K et al. Cruciferous dithiolethione-mediated coordinated induction of total cellular and mitochondrial antioxidants and phase 2 enzymes in human primary cardiomyocytes : cytoprotection against oxidative/electr. *Exp Biol Med* (Maywood). 2009 Apr;234(4):418-29. 2009.

[230] Khanna, D, et al. "Natural products as a gold mine for arthritis treatment." *Current Opinion in Pharmacology* 7, no. 3 (2007) : 344-51.

[231] Bulbus Allii Cepae. In : *WHO Monographs on Selected Medicinal Plants .* Vol. 1. Geneva, Switzerland : World Health Organization; 1999 : 5.

[232] Griffiths G, Trueman L, Crowther T, Thomas B, Smith B. Onions – a global benefit to health. *Phytother Res.* 2002;16(7):603-615.

[233] Wilson EA and Demmig-Adams B. Antioxidant, anti-inflammatory, and antimicrobial properties of garlic and onions. *Nutrition & Food Science* 2007, Vol. 37 Iss : 3, pp.178 - 183. 2007.

[234] Slimestad R, Fossen T and Vågen IM. Onions : a source of unique dietary flavonoids. *J Agric Food Chem.* 2007 Dec 12;55(25):10067-80. 2007.

[235] Effect of parsley (Petroselinum crispum) intake on urinary apigenin excretion, blood antioxidant enzymes and bio-markers for oxidative stress in human subjects," S.E. Nielsen, et al. *British Journal of Nutrition* June 1999; 81(6) : 447-55.

[236] Lee, JY, and W Park. "Anti-inflammatory effect of myristicin on RAW 264.7 macrophages stimulated with polyinosinic-polycytidylic acid."*Molecules* 16, no. 8 (2011) : 7132-42. http://www.ncbi.nlm.nih.gov/pubmed/21991618 (accessed April 10, 2012)

[237] Zhu, LH, et al. "Luteolin inhibits microglial inflammation and improves neuron survival against inflammation." *The International Journal of Neuroscience* 121, no. 6 (2011) : 329-36.

[238] Pattison, D, et al. "Vitamin C and the risk of developing inflammatory polyarthritis : prospective nested case-control study." *Annals of Rheumatic Disease* 36, no. 7 (2004) : 277-91.

[239] Hassellund, SS, et al. "Effects of anthocyanins on cardiovascular risk factors and inflammation in pre-hypertensive men : a double-blind randomized placebo-controlled crossover study." *Journal of Human Hypertension* [Epub ahead of print] (2012). http://www.ncbi.nlm. nih.gov/pubmed/22336903 (accessed April 11, 2012)

[240] Beevi, SS, LN Mangamoori, and BB Gowda. "Polyphenolics profile and antioxidant properties of Raphanus sativus L." *Natural Products Research* 26, no. 6 (2012). http://www.ncbi.nlm.nih.gov/ pubmed/21714734 (accessed April 10, 2012).

[241] Shearer MJ. The roles of vitamins D and K in bone health and osteoporosis prevention. *Proc Nutr Soc.* 1997;56(3):915-937.

[242] Booth SL. Skeletal functions of vitamin K-dependent proteins : not just for clotting anymore. *Nutr Rev.* 1997;55(7):282-284.

[243] Song W, Derito CM, Liu MK et al. Cellular antioxidant activity of common vegetables. *J Agric Food Chem.* 2010 Jun 9;58(11):6621-9. 2010.

[244] Edenharder R, Keller G, Platt KL, Unger KK. Isolation and characterization of structurally novel antimutagenic flavonoids from spinach (Spinacia oleracea). *J Agric Food Chem* 2001 Jun;49(6):2767-73 2001. PMID:12950.

[245] Jackson RD, et al. Calcium plus vitamin D supplementation and the risk of fractures. *N Engl J Med* 2006; 354(7):669-83.

[246] Dawczynski, C, et al. "Incorporation of n-3 PUFA and γ-linolenic acid in blood lipids and red blood cell lipids together with their influence on disease activity in patients with chronic inflammatory arthritis--a randomized controlled human intervention trial." *Lipids in Health and Diseases* 10, no. 130 (2011) : .

[247] Hurst, S. "Dietary fatty acids and arthritis." *Prostaglandins Leukot Essent Fatty Acids.* 82, no. 4-6 (2010) : 315-8. http://www.ncbi.nlm. nih.gov/pubmed/20189789 (accessed April 10, 2012).

[248] Xu, ZZ, and RR Ji. "Resolvins are potent analgesics for arthritic pain." *British Journal of Pharmacology* 164, no. 2 (2011) : 274-7. http://www.ncbi.nlm.nih.gov/pubmed/21418190 (accessed April 11, 2012).

[249] Aizzat, O,et al. "Modulation of oxidative stress by Chlorella vulgaris in streptozotocin (STZ) induced diabetic Sprague-Dawley rats." *Advances in Medical Sciences* 55, no. 2 (2010) : 281-8.

[250] Cherng , JY. "Beneficial effects of Chlorella-11 peptide on blocking LPS-induced macrophage activation and alleviating thermal injury-induced inflammation in rats." *International Journal of Immunopathology and Pharmacology* 23, no. 3 (2010) : 811-20. http://www.ncbi.nlm.nih.gov/pubmed/20943052 (accessed April 4, 2012).

[251] Lee HS, Choi CY, Cho C, Song Y. Attenuating effect of chlorella supplementation on oxidative stress and NFkappaB activation in peritoneal macrophages and liver of C57BL/6 mice fed on an atherogenic diet. *Biosci Biotechnol Biochem.* 2003 October 67(10):2083-90.

[252] "Anti-inflammatory effects of chlorella in chronic and acute inflammation." sunchlorella.com.   www.sunchlorella.com/assets/files/100728%20 Scientific%20Report/100728-4.PDF (accessed April 5, 2012)

[253] Zakaria, ZA, et al. "In vivo antinociceptive and anti-inflammatory activities of dried and fermented processed virgin coconut oil." *Medical Principals and Practice* 20, no. 3 (2011) : 231-6. http://www.ncbi.nlm.nih.gov/pubmed/21454992 (accessed May 8, 2012).

[254] Intahphuak, S, et al. "Anti-inflammatory, analgesic, and antipyretic activities of virgin coconut oil." http://www.ncbi.nlm.nih.gov/pubmed/2064583148, no. 2 (2010) : 151-7. http://www.ncbi.nlm.nih.gov/pubmed/20645831 (accessed May 10, 2012).

[255] Nordstrom DC, Alpha-linolenic acid in the treatment of rheumatoid arthritis. A double-blind, placebo-controlled and randomized study: flaxseed vs. safflower seed. *Rheumatology International* 1995;14:231–4, http://www.ncbi.nlm.nih.gov/pubmed/7597378, accessed May 8, 2012.

[256] Kinniry P, Amrani Y, Vachani A, Solomides CC, Arguiri E, Workman A, Carter J, Christofidou-Solomidou M. Dietary flaxseed supplementation ameliorates inflammation and oxidative tissue damage in experimental models of acute lung injury in mice. *J Nutr.* 2006 Jun;136(6):1545-51. 2006. PMID:16702319.

[257] Kremer JM. N-3 fatty acid supplements in rheumatoid arthritis. *Am J Clin Nutr.* 2000;(suppl 1):349S-351S.

[258] Griel AE, Kris-Etherton PM, Hilpert KF, Zhao G, West SG, Corwin RL. An increase in dietary n-3 fatty acids decreases a marker of bone resorption in humans. *Nutr J.* 2007 Jan 16;6:2. 2007. PMID:17227589.

[259] Goldberg RJ, Katz J. A meta-analysis of the analgesic effects of omega-3 polyunsaturated fatty acid supplementation for inflammatory joint pain. *Pain.* 2007 Feb 28; [Epub ahead of print].

[260] Ban JO, Oh JH, Kim TM et al. Anti-inflammatory and arthritic effects of thiacremonone, a novel sulfurcompound isolated from garlic via inhibition of NF-kB. *Arthritis Res Ther.* 2009; 11(5) : R145. Epub 2009 Sep 30. 2009.

[261] Williams, FM, et al. "Dietary garlic and hip osteoarthritis : evidence of a protective effect and putative mechanism of action." *BMC Musculoskeletal Disorders* 11, no. 280 (2010). http://www.ncbi.nlm.nih.gov/pubmed/21143861 (accessed April 23, 2012).

[262] Lee, HS, et al. "Inhibition of cyclooxygenase 2 expression by diallyl sulfide on joint inflammation induced by urate crystal and IL-1beta." *Osteoarthritis and Cartilage* 17, no. 1 (2009) : 91-9. http://www.ncbi.nlm.nih.gov/pubmed/ 18573668 (accessed April 17, 2012).

[263] Denisov, LN, et al. "[Garlic effectiveness in rheumatoid arthritis]." *Soviet Archives of Internal Medicine* (Terapevticheskii arkhiv) 71, no. 8 (1999) : 55-8.

[264] Srivastava KC, Mustafa T. Ginger (Zingiber officinale) in rheumatism and musculoskeletal disorders. Med Hypothesis 39(1992):342-8 1992.

[265] Wigler I, Grotto I, Caspi D, Yaron M. The effects of Zintona EC (a ginger extract) on symptomatic gonarthritis. *Osteoarthritis Cartilage.* 2003 Nov; 11(11):783-9. 2003.

[266] Srivastava KC, Mustafa T. Ginger (Zingiber officinale) and rheumatic disorders. *Med Hypothesis* 29 (1989):25-28 1989.

[267] Funk, Janet L.; Frye, Jennifer B.; Oyarzo, Janice N.; Timmermann, Barbara N. (2009). "Comparative Effects of Two Gingerol-Containing Zingiber officinale Extracts on Experimental Rheumatoid Arthritis". *Journal of Natural Products* 72 (3) : 403–7

268 Marotte, H, et al. "Green tea extract inhibits chemokine production, but up-regulates chemokine receptor expression, in rheumatoid arthritis synovial fibroblasts and rat adjuvant-induced arthritis." *Rheumatology* 49, no. 3 (2010) : 467-79. http://www.ncbi.nlm.nih.gov/pubmed/20032224 (accessed April 9, 2012).

269 Coimbra S, Castro E, Rocha-Pereira P, Rebelo I, Rocha S, Santos-Silva A. The effect of green tea in oxidative stress. *Clin Nutr.* 2006 Oct;25(5):790-6. Epub 2006 May 15. 2006. PMID:16698148.

270 Katiyar, SK, and C Raman. "Green tea : a new option for the prevention or control of osteoarthritis." *Arthritis Research and Therapy* 13, no. 4 (2011) : 121.

271 Ahmed, S. "Green tea polyphenol epigallocatechin 3-gallate in arthritis : progress and promise." *Arthritis Research and Therapy* 12, no. 2 (2010) : 208. http://www.ncbi.nlm.nih.gov/pubmed/20447316 (accessed April 18, 2012).

272 Oka, Y, et al. "Tea polyphenols inhibit rat osteoclast formation and differentiation." *Journal of Pharmacological Sciences* 118, no. 1 (2012) : 55-64. http://www.ncbi.nlm.nih.gov/pubmed/22186621 (accessed April 16, 2012).

273 Deng, R, and TJ Chow. "Hypolipidemic, antioxidant, and antiinflammatory activities of microalgae Spirulina." *Cardiovascular Therapeutics* 28, no. 4 (2010) : e33-45. http://www.ncbi.nlm.nih.gov/pubmed/20633020 (accessed April 10, 2012).

274 Romay C, Armesto J, Remirez D, et al. Antioxidant and anti-inflammatory properties of C-phycocyanin from blue-green algae. *Inflamm.Res* 1998; 47(1):36-41.

275 Remirez, D, et al. "Inhibitory effects of Spirulina in zymosan-induced arthritis in mice." *Mediators of Inflammation* 11, no. 2 (2002) : 75-9.

276 Rasool, M, et al. "Anti-inflammatory effect of Spirulina fusiformis on adjuvant-induced arthritis in mice." *Biological and Pharmaceutical Bulletin* 29, no. 12 (2006) : 2483-7.

277 Hailu, A, et al. "Associations between meat consumption and the prevalence of degenerative arthritis and soft tissue disorders in the adventist health study, California U.S.A." *Journal of Nutrition Health and Aging* Jan-Feb 10, no. 1 (2006) : 7-14. http://www.ncbi.nlm.nih.gov/pubmed/16453052 (accessed May 6, 2012).

[278] Lee, SJ, et al. "Recent developments in diet and gout." *Current Opinion in Rheumatology* 18, no. 2 (2006) : 193-8.

[279] Darlington, L., Ramsey, N. W. and Mansfield, J. R. "Placebo_Controlled, Blind Study of Dietary Manipulation Therapy in Rheumatoid Arthritis," *Lancet.* Feb 1986;8475(1):236-238.

[280] Prasad, S, et al. "Age-associated chronic diseases require age-old medicine : Role of chronic inflammation." *Preventative Medicine* Epub ahead of print (2011) :

[281] Choi, Hyon K, et al. "Purine-Rich Foods, Dairy and Protein Intake, and the Risk of Gout in Men." *The New England Journal of Medicine 350,* no. 11 (2004) : 1093-1103. http://www.nejm.org/doi/pdf/10.1056/NEJMoa035700 (accessed May 7, 2012).

[282] Lahiri, M, et al. "Modifiable risk factors for RA : prevention, better than cure?." *Rheumatology* 51, no. 3 (2012) : 499-512. http://www.ncbi.nlm.nih.gov/pubmed/22120459 (accessed May 7, 2012).

[283] Curhan, G, and HK Choi. "Soft drinks, fructose consumption, and the risk of gout in men : prospective cohort study." *British Medical Journal* 336, no. 7639 (2008) : 309-12.

[284] Aris, Aziz, and Samuel Leblanc. "Maternal and fetal exposure to pesticides associated to genetically modified foods in Eastern Townships of Quebec, Canada." *Reproductive Toxicology* 31, no. 4 (2011) : 528–533. http://www.sciencedirect.com/science/article/pii/S0890623811000566 (accessed May 8, 2012).

[285] Hutchinson D, Shepstone L, Moots R, Lear JT, Lynch MP. Heavy cigarette smoking is strongly associated with rheumatoid arthritis (RA), particularly in patients without a family history of RA. *Ann Rheum Dis.* 2001;60(3):223-227.

[286] Criswell LA, Saag KG, MilulsTR, et al. "Smoking interacts with genetic risk factors in the development of rheumatoid arthritis among older Caucasian women." *Ann Rheum Dis* 2006;65:1163–7.

[287] Zsuzsanna, Baka, et al. "Rheumatoid arthritis and smoking : putting the pieces together." *Arthritis Research and Therapy* 11, no. 238 (2009). http://arthritis-research.com/content/11/4/238 (accessed May 14, 2012).

288 Lahiri, M, et al. "Modifiable risk factors for RA : prevention, better than cure?." *Rheumatology* 51, no. 3 (2012) : 499-512. http://www.ncbi.nlm.nih.gov/pubmed/22120459 (accessed May 7, 2012).

289 Cairns , AP, and JG McVeigh. "A systematic review of the effects of dynamic exercise in rheumatoid arthritis." *Rheumatology International* 30, no. 2 (2009) : 147-58. http://www.ncbi.nlm.nih.gov/pubmed/19701638 (accessed May 14, 2012).

290 Hurkmans, E, et al. "Dynamic exercise programs (aerobic capacity and/or muscle strength training) in patients with rheumatoid arthritis."*Cochrane database of systematic reviews* (Online) 7, no. 4 (2009) : CD006853.

291 Rouster-Stevens, KA, and AR Long. "The role of exercise therapy in the management of juvenile idiopathic arthritis." *Current Opinion in Rheumatology* 22, no. 2 (2010) : 213-7.

292 Yip, YB,et al. "A 1-year follow-up of an experimental study of a self-management arthritis programme with an added exercise component of clients with osteoarthritis of the knee." *Psychology, Health & Medicine* 13, no. 4 (2008) : 402-14. http://www.ncbi.nlm.nih.gov/pubmed/18825579 (accessed May 20, 2012).

293 Berman BM, Lao L, Langenberg P, Lee WL, Gilpin AMK, Hochberg MC. Effectiveness of Acupuncture as Adjunctive Therapy in Osteoarthritis of the Knee : A Randomized, Controlled Trial. *Annals of Internal Medicine.* 2004; 141(12):901910.

294 Berman, Brian, Lixing Lao, Patricia Langenberg, Wen Lee, Adele Gilpin, and Marc Hochberg. "Effectiveness of Acupuncture as Adjunctive Therapy in Osteoarthritis of the Knee." *Annals of Internal Medicine* 141, no. 12 (2004) : 901-910. http://www.citeulike.org/user/kxl3785/article/6775144 (accessed October 5, 2012).

Section IV

21 Sample Recipes from the *Anti-Arthritis, Anti-Inflammation Cookbook – Healing through Natural Foods*

by Gary Null, Ph.D.

Here is just a small sampling of the wonderfully healthy gourmet dishes that you can enjoy on a vegan vegetarian diet. Anti-Arthritis, Anti-Inflammation Cookbook – Healing through Natural Foods *provides more than 200 tasty vegan-vegetarian recipes that will not only satisfy your palate, but will significantly reduce the amount of inflammation in your body, and help your body achieve a healthy, balanced weight. Order it today at www.essentialpublishing. org/bookstore.html*

BREAKFAST

Blueberry Apricot Oatmeal

1 cup water
¾ cup gluten-free steel cut oats
1 tablespoon chia seeds
1 teaspoon ground cinnamon
½ teaspoon ground ginger

½ cup fresh blueberries; reserve
  a few for garnish
½ cup sliced apricot
½ banana, sliced, for garnish

Bring water to a boil in a medium saucepan; add the steel cut oats, chia seeds, cinnamon, ginger, blueberries, and apricot slices. Reduce heat.

Simmer 5 to 8 minutes to desired consistency, stirring frequently.

Yield: 2 servings

Nutty Fruit Breakfast

1 cup barley, cooked
2 tablespoons barley malt
1 teaspoon ground cinnamon
1 teaspoon chia seeds
1 banana, mashed

¼ cup dried figs, chopped
½ cup red raspberries
½ cup blueberries
½ cup walnuts, chopped

Combine barley, barley malt, cinnamon, chia seeds, and mashed banana in a large bowl.

Add the figs, raspberries, blueberries, and walnuts and mix well.

Garnish with fresh fruit.

Yield: 2 servings

Quinoa Pancakes

¾ cup quinoa flour
¼ cup gluten-free rolled oats
1 tablespoon flaxseed meal,
  golden or brown
½ teaspoon baking soda
1 teaspoon baking powder

½ cup apple juice
½ cup almond milk
2 tablespoons sunflower oil
Maple syrup
½ cup raspberries

In a large bowl, mix together quinoa flour, oats, flaxseed meal, baking soda, and baking powder.

Add apple juice and almond milk and stir until smooth.

Heat the oil in a large skillet, and add pancake batter to the hot oil, creating the desired pancake size.

Cook each pancake for approximately 3 minutes or until top starts to bubble and the underside starts to brown.

Flip the pancake and cook for an additional 2 minutes or until brown.

Serve with maple syrup and raspberries.

Yield: 4 servings

APPETIZERS

Ginger Black Bean Dip

1 cup black beans, cooked
2 cloves garlic, minced
1 teaspoon ginger, minced
1 tablespoon tamari
½ chili pepper, minced

1 tablespoon cilantro, chopped
1 teaspoon toasted sesame oil
Sea salt to taste
½ teaspoon freshly ground
  black pepper

Place beans, garlic, and ginger in a food processor and purée until smooth.

Add tamari, chili, cilantro, sesame oil, salt, and pepper and pulse until well mixed.

Garnish with goji berries.

Serve with sesame bread sticks, vegetable chips, dried fruit, or fresh cut vegetables.

Yield: 6 servings

Herbed Tofu Croquettes

2 tablespoons olive oil
1 medium yellow onion, diced
2 cloves garlic, minced
1 green bell pepper, diced
3 stalks celery, diced
¼ pound mushrooms, minced
1 package firm tofu, drained
3 tablespoons flaxseed meal
¼ cup sunflower seeds
½ cup cashews, chopped

1 tablespoon tamari (soy sauce)
1 teaspoon fresh thyme, chopped
1 teaspoon fresh oregano, chopped
Sea salt to taste
½ teaspoon black pepper
½ cup wheat germ
2 tablespoons parsley, chopped, for garnish

Preheat oven to 350°.

Heat the oil in a skillet over medium-high heat and sauté onion, garlic, green pepper, and celery until the onion is translucent.

Add mushrooms and sauté for 5 minutes.

Place the tofu, sautéed vegetables, flaxseed meal, sunflower seeds, cashews, tamari, thyme, oregano, salt, and pepper in a food processor and purée until smooth.

Form the mixture into croquettes about 2 inches wide.

Place the wheat germ in a shallow bowl. Roll the croquettes in the wheat germ until well-coated and chill for 30 minutes.

Spray a baking sheet with non-stick olive oil spray, place croquettes evenly on the sheet, and bake for 10 minutes or until lightly brown.

Garnish with parsley.

Yield: 6 servings

Tahini-Broccoli Cream Dip

1 cup (approx. 8 oz.) silken tofu
½ cup tahini
2 tablespoons tamari
½ cup broccoli, chopped and
    steamed

1 tablespoon scallions, chopped
½ teaspoon freshly ground
    black pepper

Combine all the ingredients in a food processor and purée until smooth.

Serve with vegetable chips or assorted raw vegetables.

Yield: 4 servings

SOUPS

Cream of Broccoli Soup

1 tablespoon olive oil
1 yellow onion, diced
2 cloves garlic, minced
1 cup water
2 cups unsweetened almond
    milk
¼ cup cubed potatoes
½ cup broccoli florets

2 tablespoons fresh dill,
    chopped
1 teaspoon tamari
Sea salt to taste
½ teaspoon freshly ground
    black pepper
1 teaspoon paprika, for garnish
¼ cup bean sprouts, for garnish

Heat the oil in a large saucepan over medium heat and sauté onion and garlic until onion is translucent.

Add water, almond milk, potatoes, broccoli, dill, tamari, salt, and pepper and simmer over low heat for 15 minutes.

Remove the potatoes and broccoli from the soup, place in a food processor with some of the cooking liquid and purée until smooth.

Return to saucepan and stir until well blended.

Garnish with paprika and bean sprouts.

Yield: 2 servings

Italian Style Pinto Bean Soup

2 tablespoons olive oil
1 yellow onion, diced
2 cloves garlic, minced
1 stalk celery, chopped
1 red bell pepper, chopped
4 cups water
2 cups pinto beans, cooked

2 carrots, sliced
1 cup mushrooms, sliced
½ cup arugula, chopped
½ teaspoon cumin
Sea salt to taste
½ teaspoon freshly ground
  black pepper

Heat the oil in a large saucepan over medium heat and sauté the onion, garlic, celery, and red pepper until the onion is translucent.

Add water, beans, carrots, mushrooms, arugula, cumin, salt, and pepper and simmer over medium heat for 20 minutes.

Yield: 4 servings

Gary's Noodle Soup

1 tablespoon olive oil
1 yellow onion, diced
3 cloves garlic, minced
1 stalk celery, chopped
4 cups vegetable stock
1 package fresh spinach
  (10 oz.), coarsely chopped
6 stalks asparagus, cut into
  1 inch pieces

½ teaspoon cumin
3 tablespoons fresh basil,
  chopped
Sea salt to taste
¼ teaspoon freshly ground
  black pepper
Pinch cayenne
8-oz. package buckwheat
  noodles

½ cup cherry tomatoes, sliced

Heat the oil in a large saucepan over medium heat and sauté the onion, garlic, and celery until the onions are translucent.

Add vegetable stock, spinach, asparagus, cumin, basil, salt, and pepper and simmer for 10 minutes.

Add noodles and cook for an additional 10 minutes.

Garnish with cherry tomato.

Yield: 4 servings

SALADS

Artichoke and Chickpea Salad

Dressing:

2 tablespoons extra virgin
  olive oil

1 tablespoon fresh lemon juice

2 cloves garlic, minced

1 teaspoon fresh ginger, minced

Sea salt to taste

½ teaspoon freshly ground
  black pepper

Pinch cayenne

Salad:

1 cup brown rice, cooked

1 cup chickpeas, cooked

1 cup (approx. 2 • 6-oz. jars)
  marinated artichoke hearts,
  quartered

½ cup broccoli, steamed

½ cup fresh parsley, chopped

2 tablespoons fresh mint,
  chopped

2 scallions, sliced

1 tomato, chopped

½ cup fresh dill, for garnish

Whisk oil, lemon juice, garlic, ginger, salt, pepper, and cayenne together in a small bowl.

Place brown rice, chickpeas, artichoke hearts, broccoli, parsley, mint, scallions, and tomato in a salad bowl and toss with the dressing.

Garnish with dill.

Yield: 2 servings

Eggplant Salad

Dressing:

2 tablespoons olive oil
1 tablespoon lemon juice
1 clove garlic, pressed
Sea salt to taste

½ teaspoon freshly ground
   black pepper
Pinch cayenne

Whisk oil, lemon juice, garlic, salt, pepper, and cayenne together in a small bowl.

Eggplant:

2 large eggplants
½ teaspoon cumin
Sea salt to taste
½ teaspoon freshly ground
   black pepper
1 small red onion, finely chopped
3 tablespoons fresh parsley,
   chopped; reserve 1 tablespoon
   for garnish

¼ teaspoon ground marjoram
1 teaspoon fresh thyme
½ cup cherry tomatoes, halved,
   for garnish
½ cup yellow cherry tomatoes,
   halved, for garnish

Preheat oven to 350°.

Cut the eggplants in half and place on a baking sheet sprayed with non-stick olive oil.

Season the eggplants with cumin, salt, and pepper and bake for 15-20 minutes.

When the eggplants are cool enough to handle, scrape the pulp from the skin and mash the pulp in a salad bowl.

Add the red onion, parsley, marjoram, and thyme; mix well and then toss the salad with the dressing.

Garnish with parsley and the tomatoes.

Yield: 2 to 3 servings

Mellow Rice Salad

Dressing:
2 tablespoons walnut oil
1 tablespoon raw, unfiltered
  apple cider vinegar
1 clove garlic, pressed
Sea salt to taste
½ teaspoon freshly ground
  black pepper
Pinch cayenne

Salad:
1 cup brown rice, cooked
½ cup pecans, chopped
2 tablespoons fresh dill, chopped
1 yellow bell pepper, diced
1 cup cherry tomatoes, halved
1 scallion, chopped finely

Whisk oil, vinegar, garlic, salt, pepper, and cayenne together in a small bowl.

Place brown rice, pecans, dill, yellow bell pepper, tomato and scallion in a salad bowl and toss the salad with the dressing.

Yield: 2 servings

Superior Spinach Salad

Dressing:
2 tablespoons walnut oil
1 tablespoon raw, unfiltered
  apple cider vinegar
1 clove garlic, pressed
Sea salt to taste
½ teaspoon freshly ground
  black pepper
Pinch cayenne

Salad:
1 package (10 oz.) fresh
  spinach, coarsely chopped
½ cup cauliflower florets
½ avocado, diced
1 jar (6 oz.) marinated artichoke
  hearts, quartered; reserve
  half for garnish
½ cup walnuts, chopped
2 shallots, minced
¼ teaspoon oregano
¼ teaspoon sage
¼ cup micro-greens, for garnish

Whisk oil, vinegar, garlic, salt, pepper, and cayenne together in a small bowl.

Place spinach, cauliflower, avocado, artichoke hearts, walnuts, shallots, oregano, and sage in a salad bowl and toss with the dressing.

Garnish with micro-greens and artichoke hearts.

Yield: 2 servings

Entrées

Angel Hair Pasta with Mushrooms and Peas

2 tablespoons extra virgin olive oil
1 medium yellow onion, diced
2 cloves of garlic, minced
3 cups mushrooms, sliced
½ cup unsweetened almond milk
1 tablespoon fresh rosemary, chopped
1 teaspoon chia seeds
¼ cup pine nuts
1 cup fresh peas
Sea salt to taste
½ teaspoon freshly ground black pepper
1 cup sliced radicchio
⅔ cup grated vegan Parmesan cheese
3 cups angel hair pasta, cooked

Heat the oil in a large saucepan over medium heat and sauté the onion and garlic until the onion is translucent.

Add the mushrooms and sauté for another 2 minutes.

Add the almond milk, rosemary, chia seeds, pine nuts, peas, salt, and pepper and cook for 5 minutes.

Turn off the heat and add the radicchio, allowing it to steam for a minute or two.

Toss with the vegan Parmesan cheese and pasta.

Yield: 2 servings

Curried Barley with Avocado

2 tablespoons extra virgin olive oil

1 medium yellow onion, chopped

2 cloves garlic, minced

½ stalk celery, minced

½ red bell pepper, chopped

3 tablespoons sliced black olives

¼ cup cashews, chopped

¼ cup currants

1 tablespoon fresh parsley, chopped

1 teaspoon fresh cilantro, chopped

¼ cup chia seeds

2 cups barley, cooked

1 tablespoon curry powder

Sea salt to taste

½ teaspoon freshly ground black pepper

1 large ripe avocado, peeled and sliced

½ cup chives, cut into 2-inch pieces, for garnish

Heat the oil in a large saucepan over medium heat and sauté the onion, garlic, and celery until the onion is translucent.

Add the red pepper, olives, cashews, currants, parsley, cilantro, chia seeds, barley, curry powder, salt, and pepper and stir well, and until thoroughly warmed.

Garnish with chives.

Serve with sliced avocado.

Yield: 2 servings

Lentil Burgers

1 cup cooked brown lentils

¼ cup lentil sprouts

¼ cup unsalted cashews, chopped

¼ cup unsalted almonds, chopped

1 teaspoon chia seeds

1 small yellow onion, diced

2 teaspoons curry powder

2 tablespoons fresh cilantro

½ cup whole wheat bread crumbs

¼ teaspoon cayenne

Sea salt to taste

½ teaspoon freshly ground
   black pepper

Preheat oven to 425°.

Purée carrots in a food processor.

Add lentils, sprouts, cashews, almonds, chia seeds, onion, curry powder, cilantro, bread crumbs, cayenne, salt, and pepper to the food processor and purée until smooth.

Shape mixture into patties and place on an ungreased baking sheet.

Bake for 10 minutes; turn over and bake an additional 10 – 15 minutes.

Serve on sesame seed buns with lettuce and tomato.

Yield: 4 servings

Mushroom-Stuffed Tomatoes

2 large tomatoes
2 tablespoons olive oil
1 cup button mushrooms, diced
1 yellow onion, diced
2 cloves garlic, minced
1 red bell pepper, chopped
¾ cup vegan bread crumbs
3 tablespoons fresh basil,
  chopped

1 tablespoon fresh oregano,
  chopped
1 tablespoon fresh parsley,
  chopped
1 tablespoon toasted sesame
  seeds
Sea salt to taste
½ teaspoon freshly ground
  black pepper

Preheat oven to 350°.

Slice tops off tomatoes and set aside. Hollow out tomatoes leaving the skin intact. Reserve the tomato pulp and seeds.

Heat the oil in a saucepan over medium heat and sauté mushrooms until brown. Set aside.

Sauté the onion, garlic, and bell pepper until the onion is translucent.

In a small mixing bowl, combine the tomato pulp, mushrooms, sautéed vegetables, bread crumbs, basil, oregano, parsley, sesame seeds, salt, and pepper.

Fill tomatoes with mushroom stuffing; cover with tomato tops and place in a greased baking dish.

Bake for 15 – 20 minutes until golden brown.

Yield: 2 servings

Sweet and Sour Tempeh

1 tablespoon walnut oil
1 scallion, sliced
1 clove garlic, minced
½ cup water
1 cup broccoli florets
1 cup tempeh, cubed
½ cup peanuts

½ cup pineapple, cubed
3 tablespoons tamari
½ teaspoon freshly ground
   black pepper
2 tablespoons macadamia
   nuts, chopped, for garnish

Heat the oil in a skillet and sauté the scallions and garlic until tender.

Add the water, broccoli, tempeh, peanuts, pineapple, tamari, and pepper, and simmer for 10 - 15 minutes, stirring frequently.

Garnish with macadamia nuts.

Yield: 2 Servings

Desserts

RAW Berry Jello

1 cup blueberries
1 cup raspberries;
   reserve a few for garnish
1 banana, peeled and sliced

1 teaspoon maple syrup
1 teaspoon vanilla extract
¼ cup mint, for garnish

Place blueberries, raspberries, banana, maple syrup, and vanilla extract in a food processor and purée until smooth.

Pour into dessert dishes and chill.

Garnish with mint and raspberries.

Yield: 3 servings

Lemon Cherry Cake

1⅔ cups whole wheat pastry
    flour
1 tablespoon baking powder
⅓ cup ground flaxseed meal
2 tablespoons grated coconut
½ cup pineapple juice

½ cup walnut oil
2 teaspoons lemon extract
½ cup maple syrup, grade B
1 cup fresh or frozen cherries,
    pitted

Preheat oven to 350°.

Combine flour, baking powder, ground flaxseed meal, and grated coconut in a large bowl and mix well.

Combine the pineapple juice, oil, lemon extract, and syrup in a medium bowl and mix until smooth.

Fold the batter into the flour mixture and blend with an electric mixer until there are no lumps.

Add the cherries and mix until evenly distributed.

Place in a greased loaf pan and bake for 30 minutes.

The cake is done when a toothpick comes out clean after being inserted into the center.

Garnish with cherries.

Yield: 4 servings

Chocolate Pudding

2 cups rice milk
2 teaspoons agar flakes
1 cup date sugar
$\frac{2}{3}$ cup cocoa powder
1 tablespoon coconut oil

2 tablespoons arrowroot
   dissolved in 2 tablespoons
   of water
1 teaspoon vanilla extract

Place rice milk and agar flakes in a small saucepan and simmer for about 5 minutes until agar is dissolved.

Add date sugar, cocoa powder, and coconut oil and simmer for two more minutes. Remove from heat and stir in arrowroot and vanilla extract.

Place in a blender or food processor and purée until smooth. Place in dessert dishes.

Refrigerate for 1 hour, and garnish with fresh fruit.

Yield: 4 servings

Section V

Excerpt from
Death By Medicine

Introduction

Something is wrong when regulatory agencies pretend that vitamins and nutritional supplements are dangerous. Many in the media, without scientific basis, denigrate the use of supplements, yet these "vitamin critics" ignore published statistics showing that the real hazard is government-sanctioned medicine.

In many respects, however, these regulatory agencies act as their own critics. The government is not blind to its own deficiencies in healthcare delivery. The Institute of Medicine, a part of the United States National Academy of Sciences, states:

> Healthcare in the United States is not as safe as it should be...Among the problems that commonly occur during the course of providing healthcare are adverse drug events and improper transfusions, surgical injuries and wrong-site surgery, suicides, restraint-related injuries or death, falls, burns, pressure ulcers, and mistaken patient identities [all of which exact] their cost in human lives.[1]

The Institute of Medicine even refers to "the nation's epidemic of medical errors," many of which involve adverse drug reactions (ADRs). The US Food and Drug Administration (FDA) says that "ADRs are one of the leading causes of morbidity and mortality in healthcare."[2]

Archives of Internal Medicine published "A Special Article" by Curt D. Furberg, MD, Ph.D., et al., called "The FDA and Drug Safety: A Proposal for Sweeping Changes." The section "Problems with the Current System" begins: "We see eight major problems with the current system of assessment and assurance of drug safety at the FDA." The first of these says that the initial review for approval often fails to detect serious ADRs: "A study by the US General Accountability Office (GAO) concluded that 51% of all approved drugs had at least one serious ADR that was not recognized during the approval process."[3]

The irony is that safer (and less expensive) preventive alternatives are often attacked or strategically ridiculed by regulatory powers, even – or perhaps especially – when proven effective. This condescending stance toward alternatives may be fueled by their relative lack of side effects in a competitive marketplace.

Until recently, health researchers could cite only isolated statistics to make their case about the dangers of conventional medicine. No one had ever analyzed and compiled all the published literature dealing with injuries and deaths caused by government-protected medicine.

A group of researchers meticulously reviewed the statistical evidence, and their findings, included in this book, are absolutely shocking. In *Death by Medicine*, we will present compelling evidence that today's healthcare system frequently causes more harm than good.

This fully referenced book reveals a number of startling facts:
- The number of people having in-hospital, adverse reactions to prescribed drugs annually: approximately 2.2 million
- The number of unnecessary and/or inappropriate antibiotics prescribed annually: approximately 45 million per year[4, 5]
- The number of unnecessary medical and surgical procedures performed each year: 7.5 million
- The number of people unnecessarily hospitalized each year: 8.9 million

The most stunning statistic, however, is that the total number of deaths caused by conventional medicine is nearly 800,000 per year. It is now evident that the American medical system is the leading cause of death and injury in the US. By contrast, the number of deaths attributable to heart disease in 2005, the most recent year for which final data is available, is 652,091, while the number of deaths attributable to cancer is 559,312.6 "It is estimated that...565,650 men and women will die of cancer of all sites in 2008," according to the National Cancer Institute, a projected increase of 6,338 cancer deaths.[7]

We decided to publish *Death by Medicine* to call attention to the failure of the American medical system. By exposing these gruesome statistics in painstaking detail, we provide a basis for competent and compassionate medical professionals, such as the courageous Dr. David Graham, to recognize the inadequacies of today's system and at least attempt to institute meaningful reforms.

On November 18, 2004, David J. Graham, MD, MPH, Associate Director for Science and Medicine in the FDA's Office of Drug Safety, testified before the US Senate. Dr. Graham graduated from the Johns Hopkins University School of Medicine, and trained in Internal Medicine at Yale and in adult Neurology at the University of Pennsylvania. After this, he completed a three-year fellowship in pharmaco-epidemiology and a Masters in Public Health at Johns Hopkins, with a concentration in epidemiology and biostatistics.[8] His education and extensive experience qualify him to offer an expert opinion on pharmaceutical drugs.

Dr. Graham, who had spent twenty years working at the FDA, told the Senate:

> During my career, I believe I have made a real difference for the cause of patient safety. My research and efforts within FDA led to the withdrawal from the US market of Omniflox, an antibiotic that caused hemolytic anemia; Rezulin, a diabetes drug that caused acute liver failure; Fen-Phen and Redux, weight loss drugs that caused heart valve injury; and PPA (phenylpropanolamine), an over-the-counter decongestant and weight loss product that caused hemorrhagic stroke in young women.
>
> My research also led to the withdrawal from outpatient use of Trovan, an antibiotic that caused acute liver

failure and death. I also contributed to the team effort that led to the withdrawal of Lotronex, a drug for irritable bowel syndrome that causes ischemic colitis; Baycol, a cholesterol-lowering drug that caused severe muscle injury, kidney failure and death; Seldane, an antihistamine that caused heart arrhythmias and death; and Propulsid, a drug for night-time heartburn that caused heart arrhythmias and death...

I have done extensive work concerning the issue of pregnancy exposure to Accutane, a drug that is used to treat acne but can cause birth defects in some children who are exposed in utero if their mothers take the drug during the first trimester. During my career, I have recommended the market withdrawal of twelve drugs. Only two of these remain on the market today – Accutane and Arava, a drug for the treatment of rheumatoid arthritis that I and a co-worker believe causes an unacceptably high risk of acute liver failure and death.[9]

The *Los Angeles Times* reported that witnesses told the Senate panel that

Merck & Co. and the Food and Drug Administration knew before the agency approved the company's Vioxx® painkiller in 1999 that the drug could have serious adverse effects on the heart...But the FDA gave its approval without resolving the concerns, and Vioxx® was aggressively marketed to point up its pain relief qualities, not its risks.[10]

Testifying about Merck's Vioxx®, Dr. Graham states:

> Today...you, we, are faced with what may be the
> single greatest drug safety catastrophe in the
> history of this country or the history of the world.
> We are talking about a catastrophe that I strongly
> believe could have, should have, been largely or
> completely avoided. But it wasn't, and over 100,000
> Americans have paid dearly for this failure. In my
> opinion, the FDA has let the American people down,
> and sadly, betrayed a public trust.[11]

In the same way the FDA attempts to quash vitamins, they allegedly attempted to suppress scientific research, presumably to keep Vioxx® and other drugs afloat, according to Dr. Graham. "Not only did the FDA ignore known risks from Vioxx® and related drugs but...it tried to prevent Graham and others from publicizing their own research that proved the extent of these risks."[12]

When it comes to new medications, Attorney Blake Bailey observes:

> The FDA...uses the studies of the companies who
> stand to gain billions of dollars and are under
> intense pressure to beat a competing company to
> make it to the market with a similar product. Many
> of the scientists and medical doctors go to work for
> these companies after a tenure with FDA.[13]

Dr. Graham made it clear in his testimony that, throughout his career, he had only worked for the FDA, not for any companies.

> Committee Chairman Charles E. Grassley (R–Iowa)
> said he was concerned that the FDA "has a
> relationship with drug companies that is too cozy."[14]

> Sen. Jeff Bingaman (D–New Mexico) said the problem
> was within the FDA's own culture: "The culture
> within the FDA, being one where the pharmaceutical

industry, which the FDA is supposed to regulate, is seen by the FDA as its client instead.[15]

In Graham's view, the drug safety problems began in 1992 with the passage of a law aimed at getting lifesaving drugs onto the market faster. To speed up approvals, the law forced pharmaceutical companies to foot most of the bill for the review process. That left the FDA "captured by industry," says Graham. "He who pays the piper calls the tune."[16]

Edward J. Markey (D–Massachusetts) noted that a 2006 survey conducted by the Union of Concerned Scientists reported that 18.4% of FDA scientists surveyed reported that they had been asked to inappropriately exclude or alter technical information or their conclusions in an FDA scientific document.[17]

The American Society of Health-System Pharmacists reports that Graham testified "in February [2007] that, had it not been for the protection of Sen. Charles Grassley (R–Iowa), FDA would have fired him for publicly speaking out about his concerns about Vioxx® and other drugs."[18]

Dr. Graham says, "You need to weed the garden patch of drugs that aren't doing what they're supposed to do. The FDA has not been very good about that; it likes to cultivate all these weeds."[19] Dr. Graham "named five other drugs whose safety is suspect, and noted that 'the FDA as currently configured is incapable of protecting America against another Vioxx®.'"[20]

Many media sources present at the hearing, such as the *Los Angeles Times* and *Medscape Medical News,*[21] report that Graham then added, "We are virtually defenseless,"[22] but this sentence does not appear in the final transcript and may have been stricken from the record. One report begins, "The American public is 'virtually defenseless' if another medication such as Vioxx® proves to be unsafe after it is approved for sale, a government drug safety reviewer told a congressional committee."[23]

Yet the FDA crusades to prevent us from taking dandelion root.

Natural medicine is under siege, as pharmaceutical company lobbyists urge lawmakers to deprive Americans of the benefits of dietary supplements and bioidentical hormones. Drug-company front groups have launched slanderous media campaigns to discredit the value of healthy lifestyles. The FDA continues to interfere with those who offer natural products that compete with prescription drugs.

These attacks against natural medicine obscure a lethal problem that until now was buried in thousands of pages of scientific text. In response to these baseless challenges to natural medicine, here is an independent review of the quality of "government-approved" medicine. To support the bold claim that conventional medicine is America's number one killer, every count in this indictment of US medicine is validated by published, peer-reviewed scientific studies. The startling findings from this meticulous study indicate that conventional medicine is the leading cause of death in the United States.

What you are about to read is a stunning compilation of facts that documents that those who seek to abolish consumer access to natural therapies are misleading the public. Nearly 800,000 Americans die each year at the hands of government-sanctioned medicine, while the FDA and other government agencies pretend to protect the public by harassing those who offer safe alternatives.

A definitive review of medical peer-reviewed journals and government health statistics shows that American medicine frequently causes more harm than good.

Each year at least 2.2 million US hospital patients experience adverse drug reactions (ADRs) to prescribed medications.[24] The FDA acknowledges that, compared with data from the Institutes of Medicine, studies conducted on hospitalized patient populations have placed much higher estimates on the overall incidence of serious ADRs. These studies estimate that 6.7% of hospitalized patients have a serious adverse drug reaction with a fatality rate of 0.32%.[25]

If these estimates are correct, then there are more than 2,216,000 serious ADRs in hospitalized patients, causing over 106,000 deaths annually...These statistics do not include the number of ADRs that occur in ambulatory settings. Also, it is estimated that over 350,000 ADRs occur in US nursing homes each year.[26] The exact number of ADRs is not certain and is limited by methodological considerations. However, whatever the true number is, ADRs represent a significant public health problem that is, for the most part, preventable.[27]

In 1995, Dr. Richard Besser of the federal Centers for Disease Control and Prevention (CDC) estimated the number of unnecessary antibiotics prescribed annually for viral infections to be 20 million; in 2003, Dr. Besser spoke in terms of tens of millions of unnecessary antibiotics prescribed annually.[28, 29]

In 2005, Dr. Philip Tierno, director of clinical microbiology and immunology at New York University Medical Center said that each year "about 90 million antibiotic prescriptions are written and about half of those are either unnecessary or inappropriate, which is the leading cause of antibiotic resistance in America."[30]

In October 2008, Dr. Lauri Hicks, medical director of the CDC's Get Smart: Know When Antibiotics Work program, warns: "Antibiotic overuse is a serious problem and a threat to everyone's health." The CDC reports, "Upper respiratory tract infections [are] usually caused by viruses [and] can't be cured with antibiotics. Yet each year, healthcare providers in the US prescribe tens of millions of antibiotics for viral infections." Dr. Hicks explains, "Taking antibiotics when you don't need them or not as prescribed increases your risk of getting an infection later that resists antibiotic treatment."[31]

The CDC announced that to bring attention to this increasing problem, they initiated a Get Smart About Antibiotics Week in

2008, a campaign to educate the public[32] and, by implication, to sensitize physicians to the danger of over-prescribing, a practice that has been building with impunity for many years, but which can no longer be readily tolerated.

Approximately 7.5 million unnecessary medical and surgical procedures are performed annually in the US,[33, 34] while approximately 8.9 million Americans are hospitalized unnecessarily.[35-38] The Institute of Medicine estimates that nearly 100,000 patients die in hospitals each year due to medical errors. This is three times the number who die on the highways.[39]

Deaths from nosocomial infections – that is, infections that are a result of treatment in a hospital or a healthcare service unit, appearing 48 hours or more after hospital admission or within 30 days after discharge – rose from 88,000 in 1997[40, 41] to 99,000 per year in 2002.[42] According to the CDC, in American hospitals alone, healthcare-associated infections (HAIs) account for an estimated 1.7 million infections and 99,000 associated deaths each year."[43] There were:

- 33,269 HAIs among newborns in high-risk nurseries,
- 19,059 among newborns in well-baby nurseries,
- 417,946 among adults and children in ICUs, and
- 1,266,851 among adults and children outside of ICUs.

Of the 99,000 associated deaths,

- 35,967 were for pneumonia,
- 30,665 for bloodstream infections,
- 13,088 for urinary tract infections,
- 8,205 for surgical site infections, and
- 11,062 for infections of other sites.[44]

As shown in Table 1, the estimated total number of iatrogenic deaths – that is, deaths induced inadvertently by a physician or surgeon or by medical treatment or diagnostic procedures – in the US annually is at least 581,926.

It is evident that the American medical system is itself the leading cause of death and injury in the US. By comparison, approximately 652,091 Americans died of heart disease in 2005, while 559,312 died of cancer.[45]

Table 1: Estimated Annual Mortality and Cost of Medical Intervention

Condition	Deaths	Cost	Author
Hospital Adverse Drug Reactions	106,000	$3 billion	Lazarou,[47] Suh,[70] FDA[71]
Hospital Medical Errors	98,000	$2 billion	IOM,[52, 53, 54]
Hospital Bedsores	17,160	$90 billion	Xakellis,[55] Barczak,[56] Health Grades[57]
Hospital Infections	88,000	$5 billion+	CDC,[58] Weinstein,[59] MMWR[60]
Nursing Homes/Malnutrition	4,630	----------	Coalition for Nursing Home Reform[61] Consumer Affairs[62]
Outpatient Adverse Drug Reactions	199,000	77 billion	Starfield,[63, 64] Weingart[65]
Unnecessary Surgical Procedures	37,136	$30 billion	HCUP,[66, 67] Leape[68]
Surgery-Related	32,000	$9 billion	AHRQ, per Zahn and Miller[69]
Total	**581,926+**	**$215 billion+**	

The mortality costs alone exceed $215 billion a year. "Health-care costs in the United States are growing at an unsustainable rate," according to Senator Ron Wyden, who serves on the Senate's Finance Committee, Subcommittee on Healthcare.[46]

The National Coalition on Healthcare reports that annual healthcare spending in the US has been increasing two to five times the rate of inflation since 2000.[47] In 2006, Americans spent more than $2.2 trillion on healthcare.[48] Total healthcare spending was $2.4 trillion in both 2007 and 2008, or $7,900 per person, which represented 17 percent of the gross domestic product (GDP).[70] That's about 4.3 times the amount spent on national defense.[71] The total was projected to reach $3.1 trillion in 2012.[72]

The National Coalition on Healthcare further states:

It is estimated that we have spent as a nation nearly 16 trillion dollars on healthcare since 2000, but this expenditure has not resulted in demonstrably better quality of care or better patient satisfaction compared to other nations.[73]

Jason Lazarou, MSc, estimated 106,000 annual drug errors in his groundbreaking 1998 report in the Journal of the American Medical Association;[74] the Institute of Medicine estimated 98,000 annual medical errors. But if we use Dr. Lucian L. Leape's 1997 medical and drug error rate of 3 million[75] multiplied by the 14% fatality rate he used in 1994,[76] we find that the number of deaths would be increased by 216,000, for a total of 797,926 deaths annually, as shown in Table 2.

Table 2: Estimated Annual Mortality and Cost of Medical Intervention

Condition	Deaths	Cost	Reference
Hospital ADR/med error	420,000	$28 billion	Leape,[77] NPSF[78]
Hospital Bedsores	17,160	$90 billion	Xakellis,[79] Barczak,[80] Health Grades[81]
Hospital Infection	88,000	$5 billion+	CDC,[82] Weinstein,[83] MMWR[84]
Nursing Home/Malnutrition	4,630	----------	Coalition for Nursing Home Reform[85]
Outpatients	199,000	$77 billion	Starfield,[86,87] Weingart[88]
Unnecessary Procedures	37,136	$30 billion	HCUP,[89] Leape[90]
Surgery-Related	32,000	$9 billion	AHRQ*,[91]
Total	**797,926**	**$239 billion+**	

per Zahn and Miller*

"In the past, medicine was 'simple, relatively safe, and ineffective'...but today medicine is complicated...which has made it less safe, and it is still ineffective," according to Dr. Leape.[92] Emergency medicine helps many.

Unnecessary medical events, including pointless hospitalization, are important in our analysis. These events are among the most lamentable in all of medicine. They are usually preventable. Any invasive inappropriate medical procedure puts a patient at risk for an iatrogenic cascade of injuries, possibly death. Unfortunately, cause and effect go unmonitored. "At least 150 times [in the seven years between 1996 and 2003], surgeons in American hospitals have operated on the wrong arm, leg, eye or other body part."

Do not imagine that hospitals viewed as role models for research and fine clinical care are perfect. Memorial Sloan–Kettering Cancer Center in New York City "advertises that it delivers the best cancer care anywhere. But in 1995, its chief neurosurgeon operated on the wrong side of a patient's brain in part because of a mix-up in X-rays...Lapses in basic quality checks and ordinary standards of patient care led to most of the mishaps."[93]

The figures on unnecessary events represent people who are thrust into a dangerous healthcare system. Each of these 16.4 million lives is being affected in ways that could have fatal consequences. Simply entering a hospital could result in the following:

- In 16.4 million people, a 2.1% chance (affecting 344,400) of a serious adverse drug reaction[94]
- In 16.4 million people, a 5–6% chance (affecting 902,000) of acquiring a nosocomial infection[95]
- In 16.4 million people, a 4–36% chance (affecting between 656,000 and 5.9 million) of having an iatrogenic injury (medical error or adverse drug reactions)[96]
- In 16.4 million people, a 17% chance (affecting 2.8 million) of a procedure error[97]

These statistics represent a one-year time span. Working with the most conservative figures from our statistics, we project the following ten-year death rates (Table 3):

Table 3: Estimated 10-Year Death Rates from Medical Intervention

Condition	10 Year Deaths	Reference
Hospital Adverse Drug Reaction	1,060,000 +	Lazarou,[98] FDA[99]
Hospital Medical Error	980,000	IOM[100, 101, 102]
Hospital Bedsores	1,150,000	Xakellis,[103] Barczak[104]
Hospital Infection	880,000	CDC,[105] Weinstein[106]
Nursing Home/Malnutrition	1,090,000	Coalition for Nursing Home Reform[107]
Outpatients	1,990,000	Starfield,[108, 109] Weingart[110]
Unnecessary Procedures	371,360	HCUP[111]
Surgery-related	320,000	AHRQ*,[112]
Total	**7,841,360+**	

per Zahn and Miller*

Table 4: Estimated Ten-Year Unnecessary Medical Events

Condition	10 Year Deaths	Reference
Unnecessary Events	10-year Number	Iatrogenic Events
Hospitalization	89 million[113–116]	17 million
Procedures	75 million[117]	15 million
Total	**164 million**	**32 million**

Our estimated ten-year total of 7.95 million iatrogenic deaths is more than all the casualties from all the wars fought by the US throughout its entire history. Our projected figures for unnecessary medical events occurring over a ten-year period are also striking. The figures in Table 4 show that an estimated 164 million people – more than half of the total US population – receive unneeded medical treatment over the course of a decade.

References

1   Institute of Medicine, US National Academy of Sciences. November 1999. To Err Is Human: Building a Safer Health System. http://www. iom. edu/Object.File/Master/4/117/ToErr-8pager. pdf (Accessed January 25, 2009).

2   Center for Drug Evaluation and Research. U.S. Food and Drug Administration. Preventable Adverse Drug Reactions: A Focus on Drug Interactions. Last updated July 31, 2002. http:// www.fda.gov/ cder/drug/drugReactions/default. htm#ADRs:%20Prevalence%20 and%20Incidence (Accessed January 25, 2009).

3   Furberg, C. D., A. A. Levin, P. A. Gross, R. S. Shapiro, and B. L. Strom. 2006. The FDA and drug safety: a proposal for sweeping changes. *Arch Intern Med* 166 (18):1938–42.

4   Gordon S. Antibiotics still prescribed too often, includes interview with expert Dr. Philip Tierno, originally published by *Health Day News,* November 8, 2005, reprinted by *PharmDaily.* com. http:// www.pharmdaily.com/Article/1722/ Antibiotics_Still_Prescribed_ Too_Often. html?CategoryID=29 (Accessed January 25, 2009).

5   U.S. Centers for Disease Control and Prevention (CDC). It's Time to Get Smart about the Use of Antibiotics: CDC campaign aims to draw attention to the increasing problem of antibiotic resistance, (Press Release), CDC, October 2, 2008. http://www.cdc.gov/media/ pressrel/2008/ r081002.htm (Accessed January 25, 2009).

6   US National Center for Health Statistics. Deaths: final Data for 2005. *National Vital Sta.tistics Report,* vol. 56, no. 10, April 24, 2008. http:// www.cdc.gov/nchs/data/nvsr/nvsr56/ nvsr56_10.pdf (Accessed January 24, 2009).

7   National Cancer Institute, US National Institutes of Health. Cancer Statistics (projection for 2008), Surveillance, Epidemiology and End Results (SEER) Stat Fact Sheets, "based on November 2007 SEER data submission, posted to the SEER web site, 2008." http://seer. cancer. gov/statfacts/html/all.html (Accessed January 23, 2009).

8   US Senate Finance Committee. Testimony of David J. Graham, MD, MPH, November 18, 2004. http://finance.senate.gov/hearings/testimony/ 2004test/111804dgtest.pdf (Accessed January 30, 2009).

9   Ibid.

[10]   Alonso-Zaldivar, R., FDA Called 'Defenseless' Against Unsafe Drugs, *Los Angeles Times*, November 18, 2004. http://www.mcall.com/topic/la-111804vioxx_lat,0,7473253.story (Accessed January 31, 2009).

[11]   US Senate Finance Committee. Testimony of David J. Graham, MD, MPH, November 18, 2004. http://finance.senate.gov/hearings/testimony/2004test/111804dgtest.pdf (Accessed January 30, 2009).

[12]   National Coalition Against Censorship. FDA Suppressed Vioxx Studies Despite Evidence of Serious Health Risks, November 25, 2004. http:// www.ncac.org/FDA_Suppressed_Vioxx_Studies (Accessed January 30, 2009).

[13]   Bailey Esq, B., Bad medicine, *Texas Injury Law*, July 27, 2008. http://www.txinjurylawblog.com/ tags/drugs-accolate-accutane-arava-1/ (Accessed January 30, 2009).

[14]   Alonso-Zaldivar, R., "FDA Called 'Defenseless' Against Unsafe Drugs," *Los Angeles Times*, November 18, 2004. http://www.mcall.com/ topic/la-111804vioxx_lat,0,7473253.stor y (Accessed January 31, 2009).

[15]   Associated Press. F.D.A. Called 'Defenseless' Against Unsafe Drugs, *New York Times*, 18 November 2004. http://biopsychiatry.com/bigpharma/ fda.html (Accessed January 31, 2009).

[16]   *Yale Medicine.* FDA's top safety critic keeps a watchful eye on the public good, Summer 2005. http://yalemedicine.yale.edu/ym_su05/faces. html (Accessed January 31, 2009).

[17]   Young, D., Safety Experts Call for Accountability from FDA, Drug Firms. American Society of Health-System Pharmacists, March 23, 2007. http://www.ashp.org/import/News/HealthSystemPharmacyNews/newsarticle.aspx?id=2503 (Accessed January 31, 2009).

[18]   Ibid.

[19]   Loudon, Manette, interviewer. The FDA Exposed: An Interview With Dr. David Graham, the Vioxx Whistleblower, parts of this interview appear in Gary Null's documentary film, *Prescription for Disaster*, Garynull.com, August 30, 2005, reprinted by *Natural News*. http://www. naturalnews.com/011401.html (Accessed January 31, 2009).

[20]   US Senate Finance Committee. Testimony of David J. Graham, MD, MPH, November 18, 2004. http://finance.senate.gov/hearings/testimony/2004test/111804dgtest.pdf (Accessed January 30, 2009).

21 *Yale Medicine.* FDA's top safety critic keeps a watchful eye on the public good, Summer 2005. http://yalemedicine.yale.edu/ym_su05/faces. html (Accessed January 31, 2009).

22 Alonso-Zaldivar, R., FDA Called 'Defenseless' Against Unsafe Drugs, *Los Angeles Times,* November 18, 2004. http://www.mcall.com/ topic/la-111804vioxx_lat,0,7473253.story (Accessed January 31, 2009).

23 Kelly, J. Harsh criticism lobbed at FDA in Senate Vioxx hearing, *Medscape Medical News,* November 23, 2004. http://medgenmed.medscape.com/viewarticle/538021_print (Accessed January 31, 2009).

24 Lazarou, J., B. H. Pomeranz, and P. N. Corey. 1998. Incidence of adverse drug reactions in hospitalized patients: a meta-analysis of prospective studies. *JAMA* 279 (15):1200–5.

25 Ibid.

26 Gurwitz, J. H., T. S. Field, J. Avorn, D. McCormick, S. Jain, M. Eckler, M. Benser, A. C. Edmondson, and D. W. Bates. 2000. Incidence and preventability of adverse drug events in nursing homes. *Am J Med* 109 (2):87–94.

27 Center for Drug Evaluation and Research. U.S. Food and Drug Administration. Preventable Adverse Drug Reactions: A Focus on Drug Interactions. Last updated July 31, 2002. http:// www.fda.gov/cder/drug/drugReactions/default. htm#ADRs:%20Prevalence%20 and%20Incidence (Accessed January 25, 2009).

28 Rabin R. Caution about overuse of antibiotics. *Newsday.* September 18, 2003.

29 Available at: http://www.cdc.gov/drugresistance/ community/ (Accessed May 22, 2006).

30 Gordon S. Antibiotics still prescribed too often, includes interview with expert Dr. Philip Tierno, originally published by *Health Day News,* November 8, 2005, reprinted by *PharmDaily.com.* http:// www.pharmdaily.com/Article/1722/Antibiotics_Still_Prescribed_Too_Often.html?CategoryID=29 (Accessed January 25, 2009).

31 U.S. Centers for Disease Control and Prevention (CDC). It's Time to Get Smart about the Use of Antibiotics: CDC campaign aims to draw attention to the increasing problem of antibiotic resistance, (Press Release), CDC, October 2, 2008. http://www.cdc.gov/media/pressrel/2008/r081002.htm (Accessed January 25, 2009).

[32] Ibid.

[33] Available at: http://www.ahrq.gov/data/ hcup/ hcupnet.htm. (Accessed May 22, 2006).

[34] US Congressional House Subcommittee Oversight Investigation. Cost and Quality of Health Care: Unnecessary Surgery. Washington, DC: Government Printing Office; 1976. Cited in: McClelland GB, Foundation for Chiropractic Education and Research. Testimony to the Department of Veterans Affairs' Chiropractic Advisory Committee. March 25, 2003.

[35] http://www.ahrq.gov/data/ hcup/hcupnet.htm. (Accessed May 22, 2006).

[36] Siu, A. L., F. A. Sonnenberg, W. G. Manning, G. A. Goldberg, E. S. Bloomfield, J. P. Newhouse, and R. H. Brook. 1986. Inappropriate use of hospitals in a randomized trial of health insurance plans. *N Engl J Med* 315 (20):1259–66.

[37] Siu, A. L., W. G. Manning, and B. Benjamin. 1990. Patient, provider and hospital characteristics associated with inappropriate hospitalization. *Am J Public Health* 80 (10):1253–6.

[38] Eriksen, B. O., I. S. Kristiansen, E. Nord, J. F. Pape, S. M. Almdahl, A. Hensrud, and S. Jaeger. 1999. The cost of inappropriate admissions: a study of health benefits and resource utilization in a department of internal medicine. *J Intern Med* 246 (4):379–87.

[39] National Coalition on Health Care. "Did You Know?" section of home page of NCHC, 2009. http://www.nchc.org/ (Accessed January 27, 2009).

[40] Weinstein, R. A. 1998. Nosocomial infection update. *Emerg Infect Dis* 4 (3):416–20.

[41] Fourth Decennial International Conference on Nosocomial and Healthcare-Associated Infections. *Morbidity and Mortality Weekly Report.* February 25, 2000, Vol. 49, No. 7, p. 138.

[42] Centers for Disease Control and Prevention. Estimates of Healthcare-Associated Infections, last modified May 30, 2007. http://www.cdc.gov/ncidod/dhqp/hai.html (Accessed January 24, 2009).

[43] Ibid.

44   Klevens, R. Monina DDS, MPH, Jonathan R. Edwards, MS, Chesley
     L. Richards, Jr., MD, MPH, Teresa C. Horan, MPH, Robert P. Gaynes,
     MD, Daniel A. Pollock, MD, Denise M. Cardo, MD. Estimating Health
     Care-Associated Infections and Deaths in U.S. Hospitals, 2002, *Public
     Health Reports,* Volume 122, March–April 2007. http:// www.cdc.
     gov/ncidod/dhqp/pdf/hicpac/infections_deaths.pdf   (Accessed
     January 27, 2009).

45   US National Center for Health Statistics. Deaths: final Data for 2005.
     National Vital Statistics Report, vol. 56, no. 10, April 24, 2008. http://
     www.cdc.gov/nchs/data/nvsr/nvsr56/ nvsr56_10.pdf (Accessed
     January 24, 2009).

46   Wyden, Ron Senator, The Healthy Americans Act. "$2.2 trillion currently
     spent on health care in America today." http://wyden.senate.gov/ issues/
     Legislation/Healthy_Americans_Act.cfm (Accessed January 26, 2009).

47   National Coalition on Health Care. Economic Cost Fact Sheets: The Impact
     of Rising Health Care Costs on the Economy, NCHC, 2009. http:// www.
     nchc.org/facts/economic.shtml (Accessed January 27, 2009).

48   Wyden, Ron Senator, The Healthy Americans Act. "$2.2 trillion
     currently spent on health care in America today." http://wyden.
     senate.gov/   issues/Legislation/Healthy_Americans_Act.cfm
     (Accessed January 26, 2009).

49   Lazarou, J., B. H. Pomeranz, and P. N. Corey. 1998. Incidence of
     adverse drug reactions in hospitalized patients: a meta- analysis of
     prospective studies. JAMA 279 (15):1200–5.

50   Suh, D. C., B. S. Woodall, S. K. Shin, and E. R. Hermes-De Santis.
     2000. Clinical and economic impact of adverse drug reactions in
     hospitalized patients. *Ann Pharmacother* 34 (12):1373–9.

51   Center for Drug Evaluation and Research. U.S. Food and Drug
     Administration. Preventable Adverse Drug Reactions: A Focus on
     Drug Interactions. Last updated July 31, 2002. http:// www.fda.gov/
     cder/drug/drugReactions/default. htm#ADRs:%20Prevalence%20
     and%20Incidence (Accessed January 25, 2009).

52   Institute of Medicine, US National Academy of Sciences. November
     1999. To Err Is Human: Building a Safer Health System. http://www.
     iom. edu/Object.File/Master/4/117/ToErr-8pager. pdf (Accessed
     January 25, 2009).

53   Thomas, E. J., D. M. Studdert, H. R. Burstin, E. J. Orav, T. Zeena, E. J. Williams, K. M. Howard, P. C. Weiler, and T. A. Brennan. 2000. Incidence and types of adverse events and negligent care in Utah and Colorado. *Med Care* 38 (3):261–71.

54   Thomas, E. J., D. M. Studdert, J. P. Newhouse, B. I. Zbar, K. M. Howard, E. J. Williams, and T. A. Brennan. 1999. Costs of medical injuries in Utah and Colorado. *Inquiry* 36 (3):255–64.

55   Xakellis, G. C., R. Frantz, and A. Lewis. 1995. Cost of pressure ulcer prevention in long-term care. *J Am Geriatr Soc* 43 (5):496–501.

56   Barczak, C. A., R. I. Barnett, E. J. Childs, and L. M. Bosley. 1997. Fourth national pressure ulcer prevalence survey. *Adv Wound Care* 10 (4):18–26.

57   Health Grades Quality Study, Patient Safety in American Hospitals, July 2004. http:// www.healthgrades.com/media/english/pdf/ hg_patient_safety_study_final.pdf (Accessed March 3, 2009).

58   Centers for Disease Control and Prevention. Estimates of Healthcare-Associated Infections, last modified May 30, 2007. http://www.cdc.gov/ncidod/dhqp/hai.html (Accessed January 24, 2009).

59   Weinstein, R. A. 1998. Nosocomial infection update. *Emerg Infect Dis* 4 (3):416–20.

60   Fourth Decennial International Conference on Nosocomial and Healthcare-Associated Infections. *Morbidity and Mortality Weekly Report.* February 25, 2000, Vol. 49, No. 7, p. 138.

61   Starfield, B. 2000. Is US health really the best in the world? *JAMA* 284 (4):483–5.

62   Nursing Home Residents Dying of Hunger, Thirst. Consumer Affairs, November 29, 2004. http://www.consumeraffairs.com/news04/ nursing_home_neglect.html (Accessed March 4, 2009).

63   Starfield, B. 2000. Deficiencies in US medical care. *JAMA* 284 (17): 2184–5.

64   Weingart, S. N., L. Wilson R. Mc, R. W. Gibberd, and B. Harrison. 2000. Epidemiology of medical error. *West J Med* 172 (6):390–3.

65   Siu, A. L., W. G. Manning, and B. Benjamin. 1990. Patient, provider and hospital characteristics associated with inappropriate hospitalization. *Am J Public Health* 80 (10):1253–6.

66   Thomas, E. J., D. M. Studdert, J. P. Newhouse, B. I. Zbar, K. M. Howard, E. J. Williams, and T. A. Brennan. 1999. Costs of medical injuries in Utah and Colorado. *Inquiry* 36 (3):255–64.

67   Available at: http://www.ahrq.gov/news/ ress/ pr2003/injurypr. htm. (Accessed May 22, 2006).

68   Leape LL.Unnecessary surgery.*Health Serv Res.* 1989 Aug; 24 (3):351–407.

69   National Coalition on Health Care. Health Insurance Costs: Facts on the Cost of Health Insurance and Health Care, NCHC, 2009. http:// www.nchc.org/facts/cost.shtml (Accessed January 28, 2009).

70   National Coalition on Health Care. "Did You Know?" section of home page of NCHC, 2009. http://www. nchc.org/ (Accessed January 27, 2009).

71   National Coalition on Health Care. Health Insurance Costs: Facts on the Cost of Health Insurance and Health Care, NCHC, 2009. http:// www.nchc. org/facts/cost.shtml (Accessed January 28, 2009).

72   National Coalition on Health Care. "Did You Know?" section of home page of NCHC, 2009. http://www. nchc.org/ (Accessed January 27, 2009).

73   Lazarou, J., B. H. Pomeranz, and P. N. Corey. 1998. Incidence of adverse drug reactions in hospitalized patients: a meta-analysis of prospective studies. *JAMA* 279 (15):1200–5.

74   National Patient Safety Foundation. Nationwide poll on patient safety: 100 million Americans see medical mistakes directly touching them [press release]. McLean, VA: October 9, 1997.

75   Leape, L. L. 1994. Error in medicine. *JAMA* 272 (23):1851–7.

76   National Patient Safety Foundation. Nationwide poll on patient safety: 100 million Americans see medical mistakes directly touching them [press release]. McLean, VA: October 9, 1997.

77   Ibid.

78   Xakellis, G. C., R. Frantz, and A. Lewis. 1995. Cost of pressure ulcer prevention in long-term care. *J Am Geriatr Soc* 43 (5):496–501.

79   Barczak, C. A., R. I. Barnett, E. J. Childs, and L. M. Bosley. 1997. Fourth national pressure ulcer prevalence survey. *Adv Wound Care* 10 (4):18–26.

[80] Centers for Disease Control and Prevention. Estimates of Healthcare-Associated Infections, last modified May 30, 2007. http://www.cdc.gov/ncidod/dhqp/hai.html (Accessed January 24, 2009).

[81] Health Grades Quality Study, Patient Safety in American Hospitals, July 2004. http://www. healthgrades.com/media/english/pdf/hg_patient_safety_study_final.pdf (Accessed March 3, 2009).

[82] Weinstein, R. A. 1998. Nosocomial infection update. *Emerg Infect Dis* 4 (3):416–20.

[83] Fourth Decennial International Conference on Nosocomial and Healthcare-Associated Infections. *Morbidity and Mortality Weekly Report.* February 25, 2000, Vol. 49, No. 7, p. 138.

[84] Available at: http://www.cmwf.org/programs/ elders/burger_mal_386.asp. (Accessed May 22, 2006).

[85] Starfield, B. 2000. Is US health really the best in the world? *JAMA* 284 (4):483–5.

[86] Starfield, B. 2000. Deficiencies in US medical care. *JAMA* 284 (17):2184–5.

[87] Weingart, S. N., L. Wilson R. Mc, R. W. Gibberd, and B. Harrison. 2000. Epidemiology of medical error. *West J Med* 172 (6):390–3.

[88] Available at: http://www.ahrq.gov/data/ hcup/ hcupnet.htm. (Accessed May 22, 2006).

[89] Available at: http://www.ahrq.gov/news/ ress/ pr2003/injurypr.htm. (Accessed May 22, 2006).

[90] Leape LL.Unnecessary surgery. Health Serv Res. 1989 Aug; 24(3):351–407.

[91] Peck, P. Patient safety requires fundamental changes to medical systems. *Medscape Medical News,* 6 May 2004. http://www.medscape. com/viewarticle/475217 (Accessed January 28, 2009).

[92] Altman, LK. Even the elite hospitals aren't immune to errors. *New York Times,* 23 February 2003. http://query.nytimes.com/gst/fullpage.html?res= 9C0DE3D9113DF930A15751C0A9659C8B63&n= Top/Reference/Times%20Topics/People/S/Santillan,%20Jesica&scp=1&sq=Altman%20LK.%20 Even%20the%20elite%20hospitals%20 aren%E2%80%99t%20immune%20to%20 errors.%20New%20 York%20Times,%2023%20 February%202003&st=cse (Accessed January 28, 2009).

[93]   Lazarou, J., B. H. Pomeranz, and P. N. Corey. 1998. Incidence of adverse drug reactions in hospitalized patients: a meta-analysis of prospective studies. *JAMA* 279 (15):1200–5.

[94]   Weinstein, R. A. 1998. Nosocomial infection update. *Emerg Infect Dis* 4 (3):416–20.

[95]   Leape, L. L. 1994. Error in medicine. *JAMA* 272 (23):1851–7.

[96]   LaPointe, N. M., and J. G. Jollis. 2003. Medication errors in hospitalized cardiovascular patients. *Arch Intern Med* 163 (12):1461–6.

[97]   Lazarou, J., B. H. Pomeranz, and P. N. Corey. 1998. Incidence of adverse drug reactions in hospitalized patients: a meta-analysis of prospective studies. *JAMA* 279 (15):1200–5.

[98]   Institute of Medicine, US National Academy of Sciences. November 1999. To Err Is Human: Building a Safer Health System. http://www. iom. edu/Object.File/Master/4/117/ToErr-8pager. pdf (Accessed January 25, 2009).

[99]   Center for Drug Evaluation and Research.U.S.Food and Drug Administration.Preventable Adverse Drug Reactions: A Focus on Drug Interactions. Last updated July 31,2002. http://www. fda.gov/ cder/drug/drugReactions/default. htm#ADRs:%20Pr evalence%20 and%20Incidence (Accessed January 25, 2009).

[100] Thomas, E. J., D. M. Studdert, H. R. Burstin, E. J. Orav, T. Zeena, E. J. Williams, K. M. Howard, P. C. Weiler, and T. A. Brennan. 2000. Incidence and types of adverse events and negligent care in Utah and Colorado. *Med Care* 38 (3):261–71.

[101] Thomas, E. J., D. M. Studdert, J. P. Newhouse, B. I. Zbar, K. M. Howard, E. J. Williams, and T. A. Brennan. 1999. Costs of medical injuries in Utah and Colorado. *Inquiry* 36 (3):255–64.

[102] Xakellis, G. C., R. Frantz, and A. Lewis. 1995. Cost of pressure ulcer prevention in long-term care. *J Am Geriatr Soc* 43 (5):496–501.

[103] Barczak, C. A., R. I. Barnett, E. J. Childs, and L. M. Bosley. 1997. Fourth national pressure ulcer prevalence survey. *Adv Wound Care* 10 (4):18–26.

[104] Centers for Disease Control and Prevention. Estimates of Healthcare-Associated Infections, last modified May 30, 2007. http://www.cdc. gov/ncidod/dhqp/hai.html (Accessed January 24, 2009).

[105] Weinstein, R. A. 1998. Nosocomial infection update. *Emerg Infect Dis* 4 (3):416–20.

[106] Fourth Decennial International Conference on Nosocomial and Healthcare-Associated Infections. *Morbidity and Mortality Weekly Report.* February 25, 2000, Vol. 49, No. 7, p. 138.

[107] Available at: http://www.cmwf.org/programs/ elders/burger_mal_386.asp. (Accessed May 22, 2006).

[108] Starfield, B. 2000. Is US health really the best in the world? *JAMA* 284 (4):483–5.

[109] Starfield, B. 2000. Deficiencies in US medical care. *JAMA* 284 (17):2184–5.

[110] Weingart, S. N., L. Wilson R. Mc, R. W. Gibberd, and B. Harrison. 2000. Epidemiology of medical error. *West J Med* 172 (6):390–3.

[111] Available at: http://www.ahrq.gov/data/ hcup/ hcupnet.htm. (Accessed May 22, 2006).

[112] Available at: http://www.ahrq.gov/news/ ress/ pr2003/injurypr. htm. (Accessed May 22, 2006).

[113] http://www.ahrq.gov/data/ hcup/hcupnet.htm. (Accessed May 22, 2006).

[114] Siu, A. L., F. A. Sonnenberg, W. G. Manning, G. A. Goldberg, E. S. Bloomfield, J. P. Newhouse, and R. H. Brook. 1986. Inappropriate use of hospitals in a randomized trial of health insurance plans. *N Engl J Med* 315 (20):1259–66.

[115] Siu, A. L., W. G. Manning, and B. Benjamin. 1990. Patient, provider and hospital characteristics associated with inappropriate hospitalization. *Am J Public Health* 80 (10):1253–6.

[116] Eriksen, B. O., I. S. Kristiansen, E. Nord, J. F. Pape, S. M. Almdahl, A. Hensrud, and S. Jaeger. 1999. The cost of inappropriate admissions: a study of health benefits and resource utilization in a department of internal medicine. *J Intern Med* 246 (4):379–87.

[117] Available at: http://www.ahrq.gov/data/ hcup/hcupnet.htm. (Accessed May 22, 2006).

Gary's Website

GaryNull.com – Gary's official website where you can listen to his radio programs and subscribe to important updates regarding your health and the health of our nation.

Gary's Publications

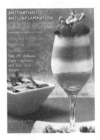

Anti-Arthritis, Anti-Inflammation Cookbook: Healing Through Natural Foods

More than 270 anti-arthritis, anti-inflammation recipes to heal conditions and diseases of inflammation, which are largely perpetuated by the high-fat, high-sugar, chemically laden Standard American Diet (S.A.D.). Prevent and reverse diseases like arthritis, cancer, diabetes and heart disease by making the delicious offerings within this book the mainstay of a new eating program...your health and life depend on it!

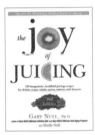

The Joy of Juicing

Get excited about juicing with the 3rd edition of this easy-to-use juice recipe book containing over 100 creative and delicious recipes for health.

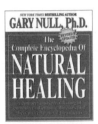

The Complete Encyclopedia of Natural Healing

This unique and reliable health reference picks up where other sources leave off, offering a comprehensive listing of some of today's most common diseases and their simple, natural, inexpensive cures.

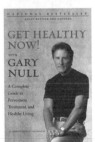

Get Healthy Now: A Complete Guide to Prevention, Treatment, and Healthy Living

This national bestseller featured on Public Television (PBS) includes research and nutritional advice for treating allergies, diabetes, PMS, andropause, and everything in-between. From healthy skin and hair to foot and leg care, this important guide features an invaluable Alternative Practitioners Guide for helping you become healthier from top to bottom, inside to out.

Gary's DVDs

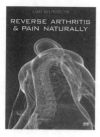

Reverse Arthritis & Pain Naturally:
A Proven Approach to an Anti-inflammatory,
Pain-free Life

This DVD takes an in-depth look at the epidemic of arthritis and chronic pain sweeping our nation today, and offers a proven lifestyle protocol for easing inflammation and pain naturally.

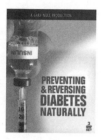

Preventing & Reversing Diabetes Naturally –
3 DVD set

Diabetes is a health crisis reaching epidemic levels in America and, sadly, more people are succumbing to this devastating disease than ever before. In this informative DVD set, Dr. Gary Null along with the world's top medical doctors, psychiatrists and psychologists will show you the latest, most powerful natural and conventional approaches for preventing and reversing diabetes, obesity, and metabolic syndrome.

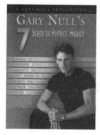

7 Steps to Perfect Health

For over three decades, Gary Null, Ph.D., has been one of the foremost advocates of alternative medicine and natural healing. Gary believes life can be lived in a manner that embraces body, mind, and spirit and that prevention is the key to healthy living. In *Seven Steps to Perfect Health,* Gary will guide you on a path toward wellness and to realizing your personal power. You will learn how to identify health-risk factors, detoxify and rebalance your system with necessary nutrients and anti-oxidants, de-stress and exercise.

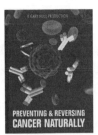

Preventing & Reversing Cancer Naturally – 2 DVD set

Cancer Can't Kill You...unless you let it! In this provocative and compelling DVD set you will learn about powerful new cancer treatments that are not taught in U.S. medical schools but are saving millions of lives in more than 180 countries worldwide, including England, France, and Germany. Arm yourself with the right information, and you will have the opportunity to avoid one of the most frightening diseases, and leading causes of death today.

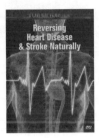

Reversing Heart Disease & Stroke Naturally

Heart disease and stroke can be prevented! There are several risk factors for both of these conditions that can be easily addressed once known. These factors can be identified with simple measurements such as waist size, and tests for C-Reactive protein, homocysteine, fibrinogen, and hemoglobin A1C levels, which can be done in your physician's office. High blood pressure, arterial and atherosclerosis, plaque and myocardial myopathy all can be reversed and prevented; learn how now!

**ESSENTIAL
PUBLISHING**

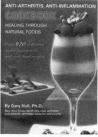

Anti-Arthritis, Anti-Inflammation Cookbook: Healing Through Natural Foods
by Gary Null, Ph.D.

This *New York Times* best-selling author brings you more than 270 anti-arthritis, anti-inflammation recipes to heal conditions and diseases of inflammation, which are largely perpetuated by the high-fat, high-sugar, chemically laden Standard American Diet (S.A.D.). Prevent and reverse diseases like arthritis, cancer, diabetes and heart disease by making the delicious offerings within this book the mainstay of a new eating program...your health and life depend on it!

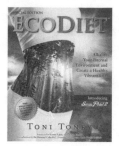

EcoDiet: Eat Clean, Go Green
by Toni Toney

Our connection to planet Earth is vaster than most of us realize. In fact, our body, like the earth, is an intricate ecosystem of interdependent organisms that depend upon one another to thrive. The balance of our ecosystem is delicate, and any disruption, such as an unsuitable food supply or a toxic overload, can damage or destroy it. In this important book, you will learn about the food choices that are creating an internal acid rain in your body – the cause of most disease – and how to restore balance and harmony.

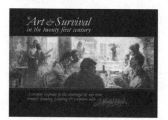

Art & Survival in the 21st Century: A creative response to the challenges of our time through drawing, painting & sculpture
by James Menzel Joseph

This art and social criticism book takes a profound look at the role of art in humanity's survival, and features over 200 exquisite and beautiful paintings and drawings of James Menzel Joseph, celebrated award-winning artist, author master art teacher, and activist.

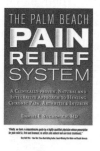

The Palm Beach Pain Relief System: A Clinically-proven, Natural and Integrative Approach to Healing Chronic Pain, Arthritis & Injury
by Daniel Nuchovich, M.D.

This comprehensive, revolutionary, proven medical treatment program utilizes natural therapies, including the whole-foods Mediterranean Diet, to overcome chronic pain. This drug-free, integrative approach is working for 90+% of patients suffering from arthritis, and other diseases of information. Avoid unnecessary surgeries and free yourself from the potentially deadly trap of unsuccessful pharmaceutical-based therapies.

ESSENTIAL PUBLISHING

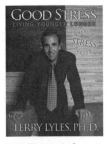

Good Stress: Living Younger Longer
by Terry Lyles, Ph.D.

Seeing stress as good is essential for achieving a youthful and vibrant life, says Dr. Terry Lyles, in this groundbreaking book inspired by years of rescue work at some the world's worst disasters: 9/11, Hurricane Katrina and the tsunami in Thailand. Dr. Lyles, known as America's Stress Doctor, implores us to see stress as a benevolent force. "If you want to live younger longer, start now by seeing stress for what it really is – a catalyst for positive growth and change.

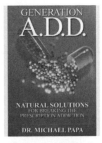

Generation A.D.D.: Natural Solutions for Breaking the Prescription Addiction
by Dr. Michael Papa

Free yourself and your children from the bonds of chemical dependency! In this timely and important book, Dr. Michael Papa urges us to explore and understand the symptoms and underlying causes of ADD/ADHD, and to choose natural solutions first, offering numerous approaches that have worked successfully with patients over the years.

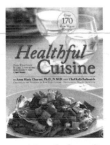

Healthful Cuisine – 2nd Edition
by Anna Maria Clement, Ph.D., N.M.D, L.N.C. and Kelly Serbonich

Learn about the superior health and nutritional benefits of raw and living foods from the world's #1 medical spa, Hippocrates Health Institute. This book contains: 150 raw and living food recipes, 40 pages of illustrated raw food preparation techniques, and more than 50 full-color photographs showing step-by-step instructions, plus tips from the experts. Making healthy raw foods has never been so easy.

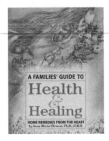

A Families Guide to Health & Healing: Home Remedies from the Heart
by Anna Maria Clement, Ph.D., N.M.D, L.N.C.

Bring healing back into the home! In this beautifully illustrated full color book, Dr. Anna Maria Clement, co-director of the world-famous Hippocrates Health Institute, show us how easy it can be to heal naturally with herbs, natural therapies, baths, flower remedies and aromatherapy. Contains more than 40 years of time-tested, clinical experience with natural healing modalities.

Index